Taking Care

A Guide for Nursing Assistants

Fifth Edition

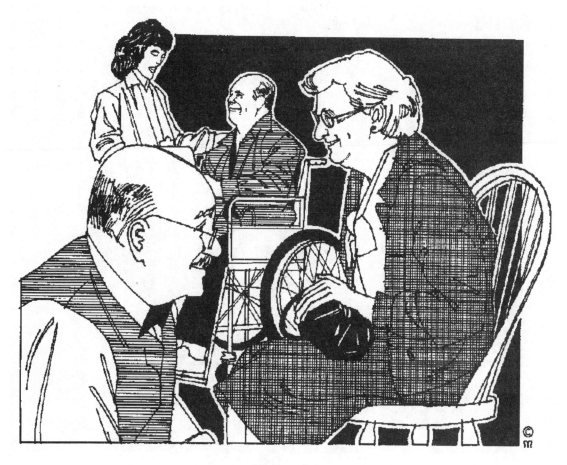

Written by
Christina Spencer, BSN, RN

About the Author...

Christina Spencer, BSN, RN, is a graduate of Seattle University with a Bachelor of Science degree in Nursing. Christina has spent much of her professional career working in long term care as a charge nurse, staff development coordinator, director of nursing and care consultant. She has been educating nursing assistants since 1980 when she started Nursing Assistant Training Institute in Seattle, Washington.

Illustrations by Travis Treser

Copyright©2014
by Christina Spencer
Updated Sept 2016

ISBN 978-0-9700845-5-2

Contents

Chapter 1

The Role of the Nursing Assistant

Learning Objectives

1. Identify three members of the nursing department.

2. Name at least three members of the restorative/rehabilitation department and describe what they do.

3. Define what abuse is and what to do if confronted with it.

4. Describe what your responsibilities are regarding confidentiality.

5. List 3 things that a nursing assistant is not allowed to do.

6. Explain what you need to do to become certified.

7. List 3 ways you can help maintain privacy for your resident.

8. Describe how you can assist a resident in voicing grievances.

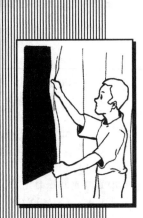

Terms to Know

mandated reporter
ethics
confidentiality
OBRA
certification
registration
need-to-know
assault
battery
slander
libel
Uniform Disciplinary Act
false imprisonment
long term care facility
abuse
neglect
geriatric

Welcome to the world of health care!

Competent, caring individuals are very much in demand and needed to make a difference in the lives of others. There are few professions where a person can make such a direct and immediate difference, hopefully to the good, in another's life. Health care can provide you with this opportunity.

You will be needed! The U.S. Bureau of Labor Statistics predicts that nursing will continue to be a career for which there will be strong demand. Opportunities currently are plentiful and will continue to increase for nursing assistants.

The following are areas where nursing assistants can find work...

- ◆ Nursing homes/long term care
- ◆ Hospitals
- ◆ Adult family homes, group homes, private homes
- ◆ Assisted living/retirement centers
- ◆ Home health care

Our population is aging quickly. In fact, people over the age of 80 represent the fastest growing population group in the U.S. today. In the year 1900 the average life expectancy was 49 years old, today it is 78 years old. That's a tremendous increase in life span within a relatively short period of time! Our elderly will in many cases need skilled care whether it's assistance in their home, in a skilled care facility (nursing or convalescent center) or in an adult family home, group home or assisted living situation. All of these will require nursing assistants. The people we take care of are called residents or clients.

The nursing assistant functions within a health care team and is a critical member of this team. In most health care settings the nursing assistant provides the majority of the hands-on care to the resident. If you ask residents who is important in their lives, they usually name their nursing assistant, frequently before other team members. They may be dependent on you for their most basic of needs, such as turning, transferring, feeding, dressing, hygiene, toileting, etc., not to mention the need for support, encouragement and love.

The average age of nursing home residents is in their mid 80's. By that age they may have outlived their spouse, children, and friends. You as their caregiver may take on even a more important role in their lives. Your competent care, touch, kind words and smile can make a tremendous difference in their life.

Becoming a Certified Nursing Assistant

In order to be **certified** the nursing assistant must pass a state approved training program that includes both practical (clinical) and classroom experience. Written and skills competency tests must be passed in order to be certified. This book is designed to present you with information necessary to develop a firm foundation of knowledge. This knowledge should help you provide compassionate and competent care and help you pass your competency test for certification.

The following are practical skills that will be expected of you as a nursing assistant.

Basic Technical skills

The nursing assistant demonstrates basic technical skills which facilitates an optimal level of functioning for the resident, recognizing individual, cultural and religious diversity.

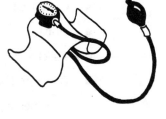

1. Takes and records vital signs.

2. Measures and records fluid and food intake and output.

3. Recognizes and reports abnormal signs and symptoms of common diseases and conditions.

4. Demonstrates sensitivity to client's emotional, social and mental health needs.

5. Makes observations of client's environment to ensure safety and comfort of client.

6. Participates in care planning and nursing reporting process.

7. Measures and records heights and weights.

Personal Care Skills

1. Assists resident with bathing

   - Bed bath

   - Shower

   - Tub

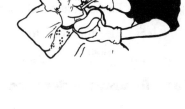

2. Assists resident with mouth care

   - Natural teeth

   - Dentures

   - Special mouth care including the unconscious resident

3. Assists with skin care

   - Decubiti prevention

   - Turning schedules

4. Assists with foot care including special needs of the diabetic resident

5. Assists with nail care

6. Assists with shampooing

7. Assists with grooming
   - Hair care
   - Shaving
   - Dressing and undressing

8. Proper perineal care

9. Provides toileting assistance
   - Bedpan
   - Commode
   - Urinal
   - Toilet
   - Bowel and bladder training program
   - Documenting toileting results

10. Assists resident with eating and hydration

11. Utilizes proper feeding techniques

Mental Health and Social Service Needs

The nursing assistant demonstrates the ability to identify the psychosocial characteristics of all clients including persons with mental retardation, mental illness, dementia, Alzheimer's disease and related disorders.

1. Modifies his/her own behavior in response to the resident's behavior.

2. Identifies adaptations necessary to accommodate the aging process

3. Provides training in, and the opportunity for, self care according to resident's capabilities.

4. Demonstrates skills supporting resident's personal choices.

5. Identifies ways to use the resident's family as a source of emotional support for the resident

Basic Restorative Services

The nursing assistant incorporates principles and skills of restorative nursing in providing nursing care.

1. Demonstrates knowledge and skill in using assistive devices in ambulation, eating and dressing.

2. Demonstrates knowledge and skill in maintenance of range of motion.

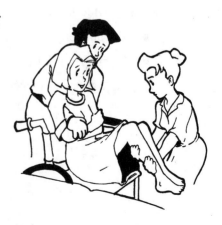

3. Demonstrates proper techniques for turning/positioning resident in bed and chair.

4. Demonstrates proper techniques for transferring residents.

5. Demonstrates knowledge about methods for meeting elimination needs of residents.

6. Demonstrates knowledge and skill for the care and use of prosthetic devices.

Clients Rights and Promotion of Independence

The nursing assistant demonstrates residents' rights and promotes independence, regardless of race, religion, lifestyle, sexual preference, disease process or ability to pay.

1. Recognizes that the resident has the right to participate in decisions about his/her care.

2. Recognizes and respects the resident's need for privacy and maintenance of confidentiality.

3. Promotes and respects the resident's right to make personal choices to accommodate their needs.

4. Reports resident's concerns.

5. Provides assistance in getting to and participating in activities.

6. Provides care of resident's possessions.

7. Provides care that maintains the client free from abuse, mistreatment or neglect; and reports any instances to appropriate facility staff.

8. Maintains the resident's environment and care through appropriate nurse assistant behavior so as to minimize the need for physical and chemical restraints.

Communication and Interpersonal Skills

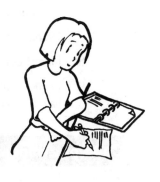

The nursing assistant uses communication skills effectively in order to function as a member of the nursing team.

1. Reads, writes, speaks and understands English at the level necessary for performing duties of the nursing assistant.

2. Listens and responds to verbal and nonverbal communication in an appropriate manner.

3. Recognizes how one's own behavior influences residents' behavior and know resources for obtaining assistance in understanding residents' behavior.

4. Makes adjustments for resident's physical or mental limitations.

5. Uses terminology accepted in the nursing facility to record and report observations and pertinent information.

6. Records and reports observations, actions, and information accurately and timely.

7. Demonstrates ability to explain policies and procedures before and during care of the resident.

Infection Control

The nursing assistant uses procedures and techniques to prevent the spread of microorganisms.

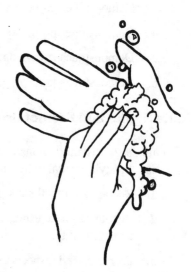

1. Uses principles of medical asepsis and demonstrates infection control techniques and standard precautions.

2. Explains how disease-causing microorganisms are spread; lists ways that HIV and Hepatitis B can spread from one person to another.

3. Demonstrates knowledge of cleaning agents and methods that destroy microorganisms on surfaces.

Safety/Emergency Procedures

The nursing assistant demonstrates the ability to identify and implement safety/emergency procedures.

1. Provides adequate ventilation, warmth, light, and quiet measures.

2. Uses measures that promote comfort, rest and sleep.

3. Promotes clean, orderly, and safe environment and equipment for the resident.

4. Identifies and utilizes measures for accident prevention.

5. Identifies and demonstrates principles of body mechanics.

6. Demonstrates proper use of protective devices in care of the resident.

7. Demonstrates knowledge of fire and disaster procedures.

8. Identifies and demonstrates principles of health and sanitation in the service of food.

9. Demonstrates the proper use and storage of cleaning agents and other potentially hazardous materials.

Code of ethics

Ethics means a code or standard of behavior that governs what a nursing assistant does on the job. This means working in accordance with proper and moral standards. Code of ethics specifically includes:

♦ Keeping promises

♦ Maintaining information of a confidential nature

♦ Being dependable, reliable and punctual

♦ Doing your very best

♦ Being respectful of resident's rights, various religions and cultures

♦ Showing caring attitude to others

- Not accepting tips

- Following directions carefully and working conscientiously to complete work assignments

- Being honest

- Doing only procedures you are trained to do

- Reporting any abuse and not engaging in any abusive behavior

- Providing for a safe and comfortable environment

- Projecting a positive, supportive attitude to resident and their family

- Maintaining pride in your profession and participating in on-going education

- Recognizing self as important member of the multi-disciplinary health care team and demonstrating sensitivity and team spirit to co-workers

- Being respectful of resident's belongings

- Keeping communication open between your supervisor and co-workers

- Accepting constructive criticisms

- Being flexible in accepting assignments

- Communicating information regarding changes in resident's condition

What Nursing Assistants Cannot Do On Their Own!

The nursing team is headed by an RN or LPN, who is responsible for assigning work to and supervising the nursing assistant. The nursing assistant works under the direction of the RN or LPN. You will take care of basic but very important needs such as hygiene, nutrition, elimination, safety and ambulation. There are some things however that a nursing assistant **cannot** do...

1. Never give any medications, prescription or over-the-counter such as aspirin, Tylenol, vitamins, etc.

2. Nasogastric tube feeding

3. Insert any tubes into body or remove from body

4. Perform any procedure that requires sterile technique, such as sterile dressing change. Nursing assistants can assist the licensed nurse doing this procedure but are not allowed to do it on their own.

5. Accept oral or telephone orders from a physician for treatments or medication.

The long term care facility

This is also known as a nursing home, skilled facility, convalescent center, or extended care facility. This facility provides care for people who are not able to take care of their own activities of daily living (ADL's), such as bathing, hygiene, dressing, toileting, ambulating (walking), etc.

A person who lives in a long-term care facility is called a resident. Some residents may remain in a skilled facility for a short period of time; others may remain in the facility for years or perhaps the rest of their lives. Many residents are **geriatric** residents (meaning older or elderly people over the age of 65) or perhaps younger people who are disabled physically or mentally. The purpose of a long-term care facility is to provide care for the resident dependent on their need, in a safe manner. The needs of the person are considered both physical and psychological. Additional rehabilitation or restorative care is provided, which works towards regaining lost skills and returning to highest level of function and independence.

Regulations guiding care

There are federal and state regulations that guide care provided to residents. The purpose of the regulations is to ensure that quality care is provided and the environment is safe for the resident. Nursing assistants as well as other health care team members must function within the framework of these regulations.

Omnibus Budget Reconciliation Act (OBRA). This is a federal law that went into effect in 1987 which guides care provided to residents in long-term care facilities. It addresses resident's rights including decision making, privacy, confidentiality, and being treated with respect and dignity. The OBRA law states that the resident has the right to be free of abuse and neglect. This includes the responsibility of facilities to thoroughly check the background of potential employees and act promptly if abuse is suspected. Nursing assistant training and testing standards were also identified in recognition of the very important role that nursing assistants play. Currently the required minimum amount of training hours nationwide is 75 hours. Some states such as Washington require more hours than the nationwide requirement. Washington State requires a minimum of 85 hours.

The health care team

Professionals providing care for the resident are members of a multi-disciplinary team. This means they have different skills, educational background, and training that focuses on various aspects of resident care. Together they meet the needs of each resident. Good communication and coordination of care is required to insure that all the needs are met. It is the nursing department that is responsible for the coordination of care.

The Nursing Department

This is the largest department in the facility and is responsible for the care provided to the residents. The RN in charge of the nursing department overall is the director of nursing (DNS or DON). Members of the nursing department are RN's, LPN's, and NAC's.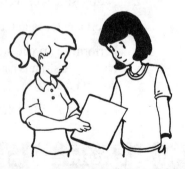

> **Registered nurse (RN)** - evaluates needs, develops a nursing diagnosis, and implements a plan of care. The RN can either provide the care directly or delegate care when appropriate. RNs provide treatment and dispense medications as prescribed by the physician. They educate patients, families, and other health team members regarding health issues.

Nurse Practitioner – RN with master's degree who does physical exams and health assessments. They may do some diagnosing and prescribing of medications and treatments.

Licensed practical nurse (LPN or LVN) - assists the RN in providing and planning care. The educational program is 12-18 months and must be followed by state board examinations.

Nursing Assistant, Certified (NAC) - assists the nurse in carrying out care for the residents. The nursing assistant works under the direction of the licensed nurse.

Restorative or rehabilitation nursing assistant - a certified nursing assistant who receives additional rehabilitation training and works specifically toward helping the resident regain skills and independence.

Other members of the health care team

The resident and his/her family - the most important members of the team!

Administrator - in charge of all the departments in the facility.

Physician, doctor (MD) - evaluates a medical problem, makes a diagnosis and prescribes treatment.

Physician Assistant (PA) - works under the direction of a physician, does some procedures and prescribes some treatments.

Dentist (DDS) - prevents and treats diseases of teeth and gums.

Dietitian (RD) - develops menus and food plans according to a physician's prescribed diet.

Food Handler/Dietary staff - prepares food according to dietary orders.

Housekeeper - maintains a clean environment.

Maintenance Worker - maintains a safe environment in good repair.

Laundry Worker - maintains clean linen, clothing, etc.

Religious staff - chaplain, minister, priest, rabbi, etc. who provide spiritual guidance.

Medical records - maintains resident's records.

Business Office Staff - responsible for payroll, paying bills, etc.

Volunteers - community comes in to provide voluntary services.

Audiologist (AD) - tests for hearing problems and prescribes hearing aids.

Podiatrist (DPM) - diagnoses and treats foot disorders.

Pharmacist (RPH) - fills physician's orders for medications, monitors for drug interactions, is an educational resource regarding medications to patients, physicians, and nursing staff.

Restorative-Rehabilitation Departments

These health care workers specialize in helping residents reach a higher level of functioning with an ultimate goal of regaining their independence and returning to their previous life.

Respiratory Therapist (RT) - assists with respiratory treatments and therapies.

Social Worker (BSW or MSW) - helps residents and their family adjust to their current situation. coordinates services available, and plans for discharge if appropriate.

Physical Therapist (RPT) - evaluates resident's needs and develops plan of care to strengthen muscles, regain mobility and ambulation.

Physical Therapy Assistant (PTA) - works under the direction of the physical therapist to assist residents with mobility needs.

Occupational Therapist (OTR) - evaluates resident's needs and develops plan of care to help the resident regain independence in activities of daily living (ADL's), such as feeding themselves, dressing themselves, etc.

Occupational Therapy Assistant (COTA) - works under the direction of the occupational therapist to help people regain independence in their ADL skills.

Speech - Language Pathologist (SLP) - works with residents with speech problems and assists residents with eating and swallowing difficulties.

Activities Director - directs and plans outings, meaningful activities, exercises, crafts, celebrations, etc.

Chain of command

This is the order of authority for the health care facility:

Administrator
⇩
Director of Nursing (DNS or DON)
⇩
Assistant Director of Nursing (ADNS or ADON)
⇩
Nursing Supervisor
⇩
Charge Nurse or Team Leader or Nurse Manager
⇩
Nursing Assistant

If you have a problem or question go to the person directly above you in the chain of command, the charge nurse. If the question cannot be resolved or answered you can proceed up the chain of command.

Health care has recently undergone many changes, putting increasing demands on nursing assistants. Today's nursing assistant needs to possess the following characteristics...

Be able to . . .

A. Communicate clearly with residents, co-workers and supervisors, both verbally and in writing

B. Question and seek clarification for anything that may seem unclear or make you feel uncertain

C. Evaluate situations and seek assistance when needed

D. Be compassionate and patient in interactions with residents even when they may be difficult and demanding

E. Be truthful and honest

F. Maintain confidentiality regarding resident/patient information

G. Manage and control your own anger in difficult and trying situations

H. Maintain good personal hygiene and a professional appearance

I. Lead a balanced life, taking care of yourself with enough rest, relaxation, good nutrition, etc., so you are able to take care of others

J. Continue learning about topics that will help you provide better patient care

K. Show a genuine interest and caring attitude toward your resident

L. Maintain an awareness and alertness to safety in the environment

M. Practice infection control techniques for the benefit of you and your resident

N. Work effectively and cooperatively as a member of the team

O. Offer constructive suggestions as to how to deal with a problem and participate in care plan meetings

P. Be reliable and arrive at work promptly as scheduled

Q. Leave your personal problems at home and focus on the resident and the work that needs to be done.

R. Be an attentive, active listener to your residents

S. Develop a trust relationship with your resident. Don't make promises you can't keep, and follow through on your promises.

T. Be non-judgmental of your residents

U. Treat residents with respect and dignity and be mindful of their need for privacy

V. Take pride in the good work you do and contributions you make to others' lives. Pat yourself on the back for a job well done

W. Take care of your residents in the same manner you would like someone taking care of you or a loved one

X. Use all your senses in making observations regarding changes in the resident or assessment of problems. Communicate your observations, concerns, etc., with your supervisor

Y. Take good care of the residents' possessions

Z. Be patient and helpful when interacting with residents' families. Remember, they may suffer guilt and grief over not being able to take care of their loved one

Personal Hygiene and Appearance

The nursing assistant needs to have excellent personal hygiene with daily baths or showers and shampoos. Use of an effective deodorant is important. Nails should be neatly trimmed in a moderately short manner so as not to scratch or injure the resident in any way. Long hair should be tied back in such a manner as to prevent hair from flying into the resident's face or food. Keep your mouth and teeth clean and breath smelling fresh. Work attire should be neat, clean and professional looking. Different facilities have different requirements, some require uniforms and some do not. Work attire should be comfortable so as to allow easy movement. Identification badges listing your name and title are required. Change or wash your clothes daily. Male nursing assistant need to shave daily or keep their beard neatly trimmed. Make sure your shoes are clean and the socks or stockings have no holes or runs in them. Cologne, if worn, should be very lightly applied since some residents may have respiratory problems or allergic reactions.

Legal Considerations

These are legal offenses that could occur. You are responsible for your own actions. If you commit any of these, you could be prosecuted.

Abuse

Abuse is intentional harming or mistreatment of a person. Abuse can be physical or verbal.

Verbal Abuse – can include spoken words, written threats or gestures.

Examples:

- ♦ Swearing at a person

- ♦ Making fun of, ridiculing or belittling a person

- ♦ Threatening a person with punishment or retaliation

- ♦ Criticizing and/or harassing a person

Physical Abuse – inflicting pain or injury

Examples:

- ♦ Striking a person with an object

- ♦ Hitting, spitting, pushing, or shoving a person

- ♦ Twisting, squeezing or pinching part of the body, or pulling hair

- ♦ Prodding or poking a person with utensils, such as a spoon or fork

- ♦ Confining a person to an area

- ♦ Sexual abuse – being forced to perform a sexual act

You are a mandated reporter! We all have the responsibility to ensure the safety and well-being of each resident. Every employee has a legal and ethical responsibility to report any actual or suspected incident of physical or financial abuse. This can include abuse of a caregiver to a resident, resident to resident, family member, visitor, volunteer or other person. Any report by the resident of abuse must immediately be passed on to your supervisor. Any witnessed or suspected criminal activity must be reported to the local police department immediately.

Negligence

Negligence is causing harm to someone due to not fulfilling duties and responsibilities. This neglect can jeopardize health, safety and welfare of a person.

Examples

- Failure to answer resident's call light or bell in reasonable period of time
- Failure to adequately supervise resident's whereabouts
- Failure to take precautionary measures such as positioning aids to prevent falls
- Failure to carry out nursing orders

Assault

Assault is a threat to do bodily harm or injury. Examples: raising a hand as if to strike someone, threatening to restrain a resident.

Battery

Battery is touching someone without permission, either violently, roughly, or forcing someone to do something they don't want to do. Restraining a person without an order from a physician can be considered battery.

Slander

Slander is verbal false statement that damages another person's reputation.

Libel

Libel is a written false statement that damages a person's reputation.

False Imprisonment

False imprisonment is unlawful restraint (actual or threatened) or restriction of a person's freedom of movement. This means restraining a resident without doctors orders and without emergency cause.

Invasion of privacy

You must treat residents with respect and insure their privacy.

Maintaining privacy

Despite living in an institution we must strive to maintain privacy for the residents. All residents, even those who seem confused or disoriented, deserve privacy. We must be mindful to preserve privacy in the following ways:

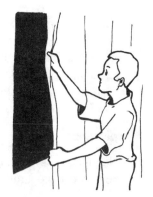

- ◆ Expose only the part of the body you are bathing or treating.

- ◆ Before giving a bed bath, pull all curtains around the bed, pull shades or drapes, close door, etc.

- ◆ Do not leave bathroom door open while resident is using bathroom.

- ◆ Knock before entering a resident's room.

- ◆ Treat their room and all personal belongings in a careful, respectful, private manner.

- ◆ Maintain confidentiality of records and personal information.

- ◆ Insure privacy to married couples.

Maintaining confidentiality

You will come across information regarding the resident that is considered **confidential** (private, secret). This information can include diagnosis, prognosis (likely out come of illness), treatment, financial status, personal and social information, etc. You should discuss the resident at the facility with other health team members, only as it pertains to their care. This discussion should only take place in a private area where other residents and visitors will not overhear it. Do not share information about a resident with friends, visitors or anyone outside the health care team. Do not discuss residents in the hallway, elevators, public restrooms, lunchrooms, resident's rooms, and other public areas. Do not discuss the resident outside the facility. It is an ethical, legal, and moral obligation to protect the resident's right to confidentiality. If anyone asks you specific questions regarding the resident and you are not sure what to say, you should refer them to your charge nurse. Anyone breaching confidentiality could possibly be taken to court, convicted and fined.

The HIPAA Privacy Rule

The Health Insurance Portability and Accountability Act (HIPAA) of 1996 established national standards for the protection of privacy of health information. The objective of the Privacy Rule is to assure that confidentiality of health information is safeguarded while allowing for access to health information needed to provide high quality health care. The HIPAA Privacy Rule applies to health plans and to any health care provider who transmits health information in <u>electronic</u> form. HIPAA is a detailed law that identifies what information can be transmitted and to whom the information can be released.

April 14, 2003 was the compliance date by which standards were implemented to protect against the misuse of health information. Civil or criminal penalties may be implemented against violators of the HIPAA law.

Resident's Bill of Rights

All resident's have rights guaranteed under the U.S. Constitution and the Bill of Rights. Federal law guarantees residents a dignified existence, self-determination, communication with and access to persons and services inside and outside the nursing home. Federal law also requires the nursing home to protect and promote the rights of each resident, including the right to exercise their rights.

The law requires each nursing home to "care for its residents in such a manner and in such an environment as will promote the maintenance or enhancement of the quality of life of each resident."

The law further requires each nursing home to "provide services and activities to attain or maintain the highest physical, mental, and psychosocial well-being of each resident in accordance with a written plan of care."

The right to safe and adequate care

Each resident has the right to receive safe and adequate care in a clean and comfortable environment.

The right to information about nursing home policies/procedures

Each resident must be informed both orally and in writing in a language the resident understands about the rights and rules governing resident conduct and of all services available and charges for such services.

The right to participate in and to determine your own plan of care

Each resident has the right to choose a personal attending physician.

Each resident is informed in advance about proposed care and treatment, about alternative choices and any changes in their health status.

Each resident may refuse care which can include but is not limited to medications, treatments, bathing, dressing, etc.

Right to notice of transfer or discharge

Each resident may be transferred or discharged out of the facility for only:

(a) medical reasons, (b) their welfare or the welfare of other residents; (c) nonpayment, unless prohibited by Medicaid; (d) upon the resident's request; or (e) the resident no longer needs the services of the nursing home.

The right to exercise rights

Residents cannot be admitted to or detained in a nursing home against their will by a guardian or anyone else.

The nursing home must encourage and assist all residents to exercise their rights as a resident and citizen.

The nursing home must inform all residents before or upon admission and during the resident's stay, on how to voice concerns.

Such concerns are to be accepted by the nursing home without interference, coercion, discrimination, or reprisal.

The right to manage financial affairs

Each resident may manage their own personal financial affairs.

Each resident may authorize the facility, in writing, to manage any part of their personal financial affairs.

The facility must have a system for full and complete accounting of personal funds.

The nursing home must have financial records available for resident's inspection.

The right to be free from abuse and restraints

Each resident has the right to be free from verbal, sexual, physical or mental abuse, corporal punishment and involuntary seclusion.

Each resident has the right to be free of any chemical or physical restraints used for purposes of discipline or convenience of staff.

Restraints may be used only with the resident's informed consent and only under a physician's written order to treat medical symptoms.

Right to privacy and respect

The nursing home must treat each resident with consideration, respect, and full recognition of their dignity and individuality.

The nursing home must provide treatment and care of personal needs in a private area.

Right to freely associate, communicate and correspond with others in private

The nursing home must give married residents the opportunity to share a room if they choose.

Each resident has the right to communicate privately by telephone or in person, with those individuals they choose.

Each resident has the right to send and receive personal mail unopened.

Each resident has the right to participate in activities such as social, religious and/or community.

Residents have the right to privately organize in the nursing home resident groups, such as resident and family councils.

Each resident has the right to receive visits from their relatives and others of their choice.

Right to maintain personal possessions

Each resident has the right to retain and use their personal possessions as space and health regulations permit.

The nursing home must have a system for safe-guarding residents' personal property.

Right to not be required to work

No resident shall be required to perform services for the nursing home.

Understanding Your Resident

Whether you work in a long term care facility, a hospital or in a resident's home, you are working with people. It, therefore, is important that you understand human beings, especially as they age and go through challenging times in their life. This chapter helps you understand your residents, including, the basic human needs everyone has, the physical changes, and the psychosocial losses associated with aging. Resident's rights will be examined so that you can be sure to preserve them in your daily interactions with your resident.

Basic Human Needs

No matter what gender, age, or background, every human being has the same basic needs. Psychologist Abraham Maslow identified these needs and called them "Hierarchy of Needs". The lowest part of the pyramid (pictured on the next page) represents the needs that are vital. The most basic of human needs is the need for food and shelter. Beyond this are other levels of needs. Residents in nursing homes may suffer from unmet needs. For example, when they are first admitted and are adjusting to new surroundings and new people, they may feel that their safety and security is threatened. Residents who do not have family and friends may suffer from lack of love and belonging. People who no longer have jobs and income may feel valueless and unproductive.

As a nursing assistant you need to understand these needs and in every interaction, strive to meet these needs. We all need to go beyond the physiological needs such as the need for food, water, etc. and recognize the emotional and psychological needs also.

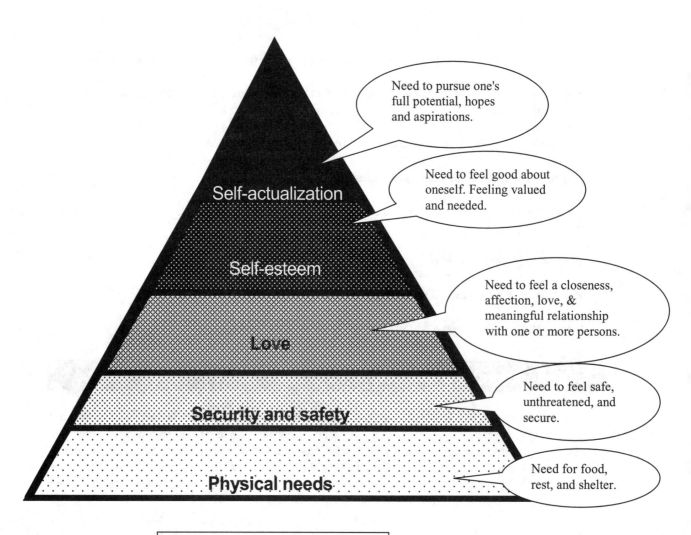

Need to pursue one's full potential, hopes and aspirations.

Need to feel good about oneself. Feeling valued and needed.

Need to feel a closeness, affection, love, & meaningful relationship with one or more persons.

Need to feel safe, unthreatened, and secure.

Need for food, rest, and shelter.

Self-actualization

Self-esteem

Love

Security and safety

Physical needs

Hierarchy of Needs

Ways We Can Meet Resident's Needs

Physiological Needs

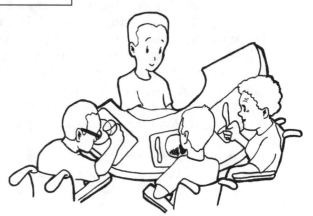

- ◆ Provide fluids.

- ◆ Assist with eating.

- ◆ Position properly for good air exchange.

- ◆ Provide an environment conducive for sleep that is quiet, comfortable and the appropriate room temperature.

- ◆ Realize that residents, no matter what age, are sexual beings and may express sexuality. Provide an environment where this can be done appropriately, i.e., provide privacy, and do not be judgmental.

- ◆ Make sure the environment is comfortable and pleasant.

Safety and Security Needs

♦ Make sure that the environment is safe and free of hazards.

♦ Use standard precautions in all interactions as a means of controlling infection.

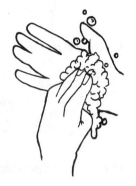

♦ Observe and remove combative residents who may be a threat.

♦ Make sure there is no clutter or obstacles to safe ambulation.

♦ Respond promptly to call light and all resident's needs.

♦ Make sure all equipment is in good repair.

♦ Observe smoking policy of facility and watch for fire hazards.

♦ Assist for safe ambulation.

Need for Belonging and Love

♦ Treat residents with respect and dignity.

♦ Encourage resident's participation in the resident's council.

♦ Provide avenues for voicing grievances.

♦ Offer the resident choices and decision making opportunities.

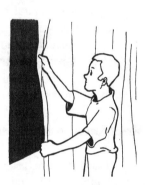

♦ Provide for privacy.

♦ Knock on the door before entering.

♦ Explain what you are about to do.

♦ Treat the resident's belongings with care and respect.

♦ Treat the family, friends, and visitors with respect.

♦ Use appropriate touch, hugs, and smiles to convey a caring attitude.

♦ Listen to the resident's concerns, feelings, and suggestions.

Self Esteem Needs

♦ Encourage independence and offer decision making opportunities.

♦ Praise progress even if minor.

♦ Accentuate the positive.

♦ Express an interest in the resident and care enough to learn more about them.

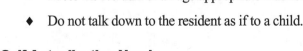

♦ Dress the resident in an age appropriate manner.

♦ Do not talk down to the resident as if to a child.

Self Actualization Needs

♦ Respect the religious beliefs of the resident even if they are not your own.

♦ If the resident wishes, help get them ready for church services.

- ◆ Report the resident's request for clergy.

- ◆ Find out what interests or talents the resident has and encourage participation in this if possible.

Unmet Needs

Individuals are affected adversely whenever basic needs are not met. They are said to be in stress. Stress may be physical, emotional, mental, social, or a combination of these. Common reactions to stress when basic needs are not met are fear, anger, anxiety, depression, aggression, regression, discouragement, and physical ailments.

Cultural Differences

You will be taking care of residents who come from diverse cultural backgrounds. What we mean by culture is ethnic background, nationality, religion, and social group. This social group usually shares customs, values and beliefs. They frequently practice the same religion and uphold the same traditions.

A person's cultural background may determine the resident's attitude to health, family, life and death. Cultural expression helps a person feel more comfortable in their surroundings. This expression can be in the form of ethnic music, art, pictures, food or participating in holiday celebrations. Some attitudes or expressions may seem strange or unusual but we must remain respectful and non-judgmental. In fact, we can learn and broaden our horizons by understanding other cultures.

Religion and the Resident

As a nursing assistant you will come across many residents who practice different and diverse religions. It is a right of the resident to participate in religious activities of their choice. Religious beliefs can provide support, re-assurance and hope to residents during difficult times. Expression and participation of religious beliefs is to be encouraged and supported.

The nursing assistant can help the resident meet their religious needs by...

- ◆ Being respectful of religious differences.

- ◆ Knowing religious preference of the resident and get them ready for participation in scheduled religious activities if they wish to do so.

- ◆ Notifying the charge nurse if the resident requests a visit by their clergy.

- ◆ Learning as much as you can about various religions and their belief systems.

- ◆ Not engaging in heated debates on doctrine and theology.

- ◆ Praying with the resident if they request it, if you are comfortable in doing so.

Sexuality and the Resident

Sexuality is a part of every human being, no matter what age or what disability they may have. What is meant by sexuality is not only the sex act but also a need for intimacy, closeness, love, belonging, and affection. In fact the need for feeling loved and wanted may be even greater than before because at this point in their life, the resident has suffered many losses.

Nervous System

This system coordinates body functions and allows the body to see, hear, smell, taste, touch and interact with the environment. The brain, spinal cord and nerves make up the nervous system.

Aging Changes...

1. Neuron cells (nerve cells) that transmit messages throughout the body decrease. This causes slowing down of responses and reflexes. A person therefore has a longer response time.

2. Nerve endings in the skin are not as sensitive resulting in decreased sensitivity to pain. (Pain is an important indicator that something is wrong.)

3. Sleep pattern changes, with shorter sleep time.

4. Short term memory impairment with more difficulty remembering recent names, phone numbers, etc. This is variable from person to person.

Nursing Measures...

- The resident may not be able to tell you that he/she has an open sore, wound, burn, or cut, etc., therefore you must inspect his/her skin condition, etc. Be aware of the resident possibly exposing self to dangerous situations and not reacting because of little or no pain.

- Safety precautions are a consideration since the resident may take longer to respond to danger. It may take the resident longer to react to directions. Give the resident adequate time to respond and do not "overload" with unnecessarily long instructions.

Common Disorders: Parkinson's disease, Alzheimer's disease, other dementias, seizures, epilepsy, brain or spinal cord injuries, multiple sclerosis.

Urinary System

This system cleans the blood of waste products, manufactures and excretes urine from the body and maintains water balance in the body. The kidneys, ureters, bladder, urethra and meatus make up the urinary system.

Aging Changes...

1. Waste products build up in the body because the kidneys are less effective in filtering out poisons and because there is slowed circulation to the kidneys.

2. Decreased bladder capacity and muscle tone resulting in an inability to hold urine.

3. Inability to empty bladder completely. (Residual urine in bladder may result in urinary tract infection.)

4. Men may have enlarged prostate glands making it difficult to empty the bladder or start urination.

Nursing Measures...

- Be aware that the resident may be incontinent or dribble urine at times. Insure good skin care by giving peri-care after each incontinence incidence. Safety precautions to keep floors dry and prevent falls.

- Position the resident in normal sitting (female) or standing (male) position to insure complete urinary evacuation.

- Be alert for signs of urinary tract infection; pain and burning on urination, feeling of frequency of urination, foul smelling cloudy urine, etc.

Common Disorders: Urinary tract infection (UTI), urinary incontinence, enlarged prostate in men

Special Senses

This system includes sight, hearing, touch, taste, and smell.

Aging Changes...

Sight   Increased problem with farsightedness

Decreased peripheral vision

Pastel colors are more difficult to see

Depth perception and distance judgment problems

Difficulty adjusting to glare

Eyes take longer to adjust to light

Hearing   Decreased hearing, especially of high-pitched sounds

Touch   Decrease in sensitivity of receptors in the skin affecting sense of touch

Smell   Decreased sense of smell

Taste   Foods taste more bland

Nursing Measures...

- Safety precautions are of utmost importance, since the resident is not able to "experience" the environment to the fullest.

- Reality orientation to compensate for decreased sensory input.

- Use bright colors in resident's surroundings.

- Speak to the resident in a clear, low-pitched voice while facing them.

- Observe resident's skin condition yourself; do not wait for resident to report cuts, wounds, etc., because he/she may not feel pain acutely.

- Season foods; serve attractive foods to stimulate appetite.

Common Disorders: glaucoma, cataracts, diabetic retinopathy, macular degeneration, hearing loss, ringing in the ears (tinnitis), dizziness

Integumentary System

This system provides a protective covering for the body, helps regulate body temperature and prevents loss of water. It includes skin, sweat glands, oil glands, hair, fingernails, and toenails.

Aging Changes...

1. Skin is fragile & tears easily.

2. Skin may be dry due to less active sweat and oil glands

3. Fingernails become thick and hard

4. Skin wrinkles

5. Person feels cold more due to loss of fatty layer between skin and bone which provides insulation.

6. Hair thins, becomes coarser & grays.

7. Toenails usually are thick & hard to trim.

8. Skin is less able to regulate body temperature.

Nursing Measures...

- Handle resident carefully to avoid injury to the skin.

- Insure adequate fluid intake.

- Use lotion. Rinse and thoroughly dry skin after using soap and water.

- Special toenail and nail care or podiatric care if needed.

- Check to see if resident is warm enough and provide extra warmth as needed.

Common Disorders: decubitus ulcer, diabetic ulcers, rashes, skin infections

Musculoskeletal System

This system is made up of muscles, bones, ligaments, tendons and cartilage. It allows body movement, maintains posture and protects the internal body organs.

Aging Changes...

1. Decrease of muscle strength and agility due to atrophy and weakness

2. Bones are less dense and become brittle with increased risk of fractures

3. Proportion of muscle fibers to fat cells is decreased and muscles lose their tone

4. Joints become stiff making movement difficult

5. Compression of the vertebral column resulting in stooped posture and loss of height

Nursing Measures...

- Residents may need extra assistance in ambulation, ADL's, etc.

- Insure resident's safety since resident may be weak, less agile and unable to respond quickly to an unsafe situation.

- Make the environment as safe as possible to prevent falls.

- Encourage muscle strengthening exercises and mobility to maintain strength.

- Range of motion exercises to prevent contractures.

Common Disorders: fractures, arthritis, osteoporosis, contractures

Endocrine System

This system includes glands that secrete hormones which regulate body functioning. These glands are the pituitary, adrenal, thyroid, pancreas, parathyroid, gonads, and thymus.

1. There is a general decrease in hormones produced including estrogen, progesterone, and insulin.

2. As hormone levels decrease, the ability to regulate body activities decreases.

Common Disorders: diabetes mellitus, hypothyroidism, hyperthyroidism

Reproductive System

In the female this includes, ovaries, fallopian tubes, uterus, vagina, and breasts. In the male this includes the testes, scrotum, penis, and prostate gland.

1. There is a decrease in estrogen in the female leading to menopause. Additionally, there is drying and thinning of the vaginal walls. Fertility ends with menopause.

2. Hormone level changes in men with decrease in sperm. The prostate gland enlarges creating pressure on the urethra.

Psychosocial Aging Changes and Losses

As a person grows older there are psychosocial changes and losses. The term "psycho" means emotional or mental and "social" means way of relating to people.

The following are some psychosocial changes a person may go through.

Retirement from work - This is sometimes accompanied by loss of identity, loss of self worth and loss of sense of productivity. This is especially traumatic for the person who may not have developed other interests and have much of their self image intertwined with their job.

Decreased income - A drop in income may occur with retirement. This may cause a drop in living standards and options in later years. Decreased finances may require change in housing, such as making it necessary to sell a home.

Increased health problems - This is more likely as one ages with possible disabilities that can affect whether one can drive, where they can live, and whether they can maintain their independence. Their comfort level and quality of life may be affected. Health problems or disabilities may lead to social isolation.

Possible death of spouse - The person may need to deal with grief related to the loss of their spouse. The older the person gets, the more likely that they will outlive their spouse and maybe even their children and friends.

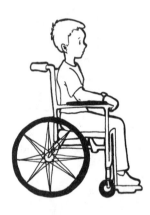

Increased isolation - Being a very mobile society in the US, frequently family members live out of town. The person therefore may not have anyone locally to call on for assistance or just for company. Health problems or disabilities may effect how people ambulate and move about. Impaired ambulation may contribute to being isolated from others.

Change in housing - They may need to sell and/or move from their home due to finances or increasing difficulties in taking care of a large home or apartment. Moving can be traumatic especially having to get rid of many belongings with sentimental attachments. Moving requires quite an adjustment to a new community and new neighbors.

Workplace Violence

Workplace violence can occur in all workplace settings. Occupational Safety and Health Administration (OSHA) reports that more assaults occur in health care settings than in other work environments. Whether you work in a hospital, a nursing home, in a private home, or assisted living, you are going to be working with patients and have exposure to visitors and family members. Some of these people may have unstable psychiatric conditions, abuse alcohol or drugs, or have dementia. They may exhibit anger, frustration, poor impulse control, and on occasion may be violent. The person may be in pain, suffered recent losses, such as loss of health and independence, or have been informed of a terminal diagnosis or poor prognosis. They may be angry at the world and therefore act rudely, impatiently, may be abusive, or even act violently to those around them.

The special challenge to health care workers is to understand why this behavior is occurring and act with compassion while still maintaining safety to self, the patient, and others. If the person becomes agitated or aggressive, speak to them in a calm manner without raising your voice. Be aware of what you appear like to them. You want to appear relaxed and non-threatening. Do not hover over them, touch or scowl at them. Stand back so they cannot hit, kick, or pinch you. Listen to them without interrupting them. If this does not work, or is inappropriate for that situation, you

9. The most basic of human needs as described by Abraham Maslow is...

    a. physical
    b. self esteem and respect
    c. self actualization
    d. safety

10. If you witness abuse, you should...

    a. tell the person doing it not to do it
    b. notify your charge nurse immediately
    c. tell the resident to ignore it
    d. hope it will stop

Describe at least one aging change related to the following.

11. cardiovascular system

    _____

12. digestive system

    _____

13. muscular system

    _____

14. respiratory system

    _____

15. urinary system

    _____

16. vision

    _____

17. hearing

    _____

18. integumentary system (skin)

    _____

19. Explain what you can do for the resident who has poor circulation.

    _____

20. Describe 3 psychosocial losses a person may suffer associated with aging.

    _____

    _____

    _____

Chapter 3

Communication, Observations, and the Medical Record

Learning Objectives

1. Describe three things to remember when communicating with each of the following; the hearing impaired, the confused resident, the aphasic resident.

2. Describe at least 5 observations that should be reported to the nurse regarding a change in the resident's condition.

3. List 3 things to remember about documentation on the medical record.

4. Identify 4 components or contents of the medical record.

5. Describe how to store a hearing aid and how to put it in for the resident.

6. Explain what verbal and non-verbal communication is.

7. Explain the difference between subjective and objective reporting.

8. Describe possible signs indicating that a resident is in pain.

9. Demonstrate ways of documenting pain.

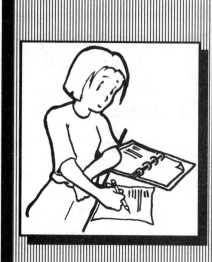

Terms to Know

documentation
verbal communication
non-verbal communication
medical record
aphasia
subjective reporting
objective reporting

COMMUNICATION

Since health care is a people-oriented profession, communication is very important. You will need to communicate effectively with your supervisors, your co-workers, your residents and their family and visitors. What makes communication more challenging is that you will need to communicate with the confused and disoriented resident, the hard-of-hearing resident and residents who have aphasia (not able to understand speech or not being able to speak effectively). Understanding good communication therefore is very important.

Ten Commandments of Good Communication

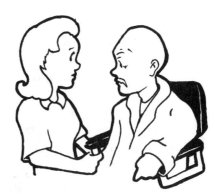

1. Be aware of your body language, facial expressions and how you appear to the resident. This is important for every resident but especially for the confused resident who relies more on non-verbal communication. A person who appears relaxed, friendly, non-threatening and not rushed, can more quickly put the resident at ease. When the resident is at ease, communication can flow more easily.

2. Get the resident's attention. Get down to their level, which may mean that you bend, stoop or sit down and make eye contact while speaking or listening.

3. Call them by their desired name. Many people prefer to be called by a title or Mr. or Mrs. or Miss. Abide by their preferences.

4. Look for non-verbal cues of the resident while they're speaking, for example, do they seem upset, are they frowning, smiling, etc.? Take in the whole message, verbal and non-verbal.

5. Be an active listener, that is listen carefully and allow resident adequate time to express themselves. Paraphrase, that is, repeat back to the resident what you understood them to say. This is to check if your understanding is correct.

6. Be patient, do not rush the resident. Show the resident that you care about them, their needs and opinions.

7. Speak in a clear, concise manner. Do not talk to an adult as if to a child.

8. Don't jump to conclusions or make assumptions. Listen to what the resident is saying.

9. Ask questions if you do not understand and give the resident feedback about what you do understand or don't understand.

10. Don't be judgmental. Allow the resident their opinions and treat them respectfully.

Communicating with the Non-English Speaking Resident

As a nursing assistant you will be working with and helping people from various backgrounds, cultures and walks of life. These residents may have different cultures and religious traditions, values and behavior patterns than yours. It is very important at all times to be understanding, accepting and respectful of others beliefs. Different customs and languages may seem strange to you but remember that the other person may perceive you the same way.

Foreign born residents may have difficulty understanding our language and customs. To help put them at ease and allow them the ability to communicate, the following may be helpful.

♦ Write out key phrases phonetically from the resident's language into English. This can be obtained from the resident's family or translator. This can be posted at the bedside for other caregivers to use also. Some phrases you could use are "Are you hungry?", "Are you cold?", "I'm going to help you with your bath". Think about other phrases that are crucial also.

♦ Use pictures to communicate information such as pictures of a sweater, glass of water, blanket, etc.

♦ Use body language, gestures and facial expressions to convey information.

♦ Use simple words and phrases and re-phrase if necessary.

♦ Check to see if the resident understood.

♦ Take time to learn more about the resident and their customs.

Blocks to Communication

Ideal communication is when the sender (the speaker) sends the message to the receiver (the listener), and the receiver understands it the way it was intended. There are blocks to communication you may encounter however.

♦ Physical blocks can be a foreign language that is not understandable to one person, inability to see or hear, or a speech impediment.

♦ Mental blocks can be an inability to interpret messages due to a stroke or brain injury or dementia.

♦ Emotional blocks can be fear, anger, hostility or delusional thinking that prevents absorbing the message.

These blocks can make communication either more difficult or prevent communication from occurring at all.

Different Types Of Communication

Verbal Communication

This can include written or spoken messages that use words.

Nonverbal Communication

This is any message sent without words. This can include body posture, eye contact, smiles, gestures, facial expressions, frowns (body language). Non-verbal communication can send very powerful messages to the resident, so be aware of how you present yourself to the resident and how the resident perceives you. When approaching the resident, do you appear friendly and helpful? Does your tone of voice, body language, and the words you use put your resident at ease or make them uncomfortable and fearful? Do you appear approachable?

Touch

A very important part of non-verbal communication is touch. It can convey a feeling of affection, caring, love and support. This can include a hug, holding or touching hands, or a pat on the shoulder. Being touched in one of the above ways can help a resident feel someone cares about them and that they are not alone. Different people, however, have different comfort levels regarding touch. Some want and welcome touch and others are less comfortable with it. This can be due to their cultural background or how they were brought up. Some people do not want their "personal space" invaded. Do use touch in the appropriate ways listed above. If you do observe that the resident does not seem comfortable with this, you can alter your behavior accordingly.

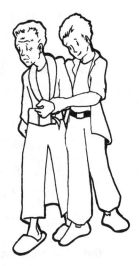

The Importance of Good Communication Skills

Communication between you and the resident, you and your co-worker and you and your supervisor is vital! You must understand and be understood in order to do your work successfully. You must understand and follow directions carefully. Remember, when you are taking care of residents it is important to speak to them, explain what you are doing, listen to them and respond appropriately.

Maintaining verbal and non-verbal communication should be an integral part of the care for the geriatric resident. The need to communicate is even more important to the residents experiencing sensory impairments such as hearing loss, etc. Communication will stimulate the remaining senses, develop trust and promote self-awareness.

Setting the Tone of Communication

1. Think about how you are presenting yourself.

2. Try a calm, gentle, matter-of-fact approach.

3. Use a non-demanding approach. Try humor, cajoling, cheerfulness.

4. Try using touch to help convey your message.

5. Begin your conversation socially.

When You Are Having Trouble Being Understood

1. Be sure you are allowing enough time.

2. Try demonstrating visually what you are saying.

3. Think about the complexity of what you are saying.

4. Try a hug and a change of subject.

When You Are Having Trouble Understanding

1. Listen actively and carefully to what the person its trying to say.

2. Focus on a word or phrase that makes sense.

3. Respond to the emotional tone of the statement.

4. Try to stay calm and be patient.

5. Ask family members about possible meanings for words, names or phrases you do not understand.

Things Not To Do

1. Don't argue with the person.

2. Don't order the person around.

3. Don't tell the person what he or she can't do.

4. Don't be condescending ("talking down" to a person).

5. Don't ask a lot of direct questions that rely on a good memory.

6. Don't talk about people in front of them.

When Verbal Communication Fails

1. Try distracting the person.

2. Ignore a verbal outburst if you can't think of a positive response.

3. Try other forms of communication.

Challenging Communication

Tips For Talking To The Hearing Impaired

1. Speak in a moderately loud voice.

2. Speak as clearly and accurately as possible.

3. Get the persons attention before you start talking to him or her.

4. Face the person directly on the same level whenever possible, making eye contact.

5. Keep your hands away from your face while talking. Make sure your face can be seen by good lighting and avoid glare.

6. Reduce or eliminate background noise while carrying out a conversation.

7. Do not turn away in the middle of the sentence.

8. Recognize that hearing impaired people hear and understand less when they are ill or tired.

9. For someone who is totally deaf, communication can occur by lip reading if the resident is able to do that. Communication can also take place by the written word.

Often we take the self-respect and dignity from our residents without meaning to do it. Here are some of the ways. Can you mention others?

1. Talking about the person in his presence as if they were not in the room.

2. Addressing a resident by his first name (or pet name) without getting permission to do so.

3. Leaving the door open when the resident is in the shower or toilet or being given a backrub.

4. Doing something to a person or for a person without first explaining what is to be done or asking permission to do it.

5. Talking "baby talk" to a resident.

6. Talking to the resident as though he or she were a small child.

7. Using the pronoun "we" when you really mean "you."

8. Failing to consult the resident in matters concerning his or her care.

9. Failing to accept the resident as he is now, wanting him to be something he doesn't want to be or cannot be.

10. Doing things for the resident that he or she clearly can do for himself or herself if given time.

11. Speaking a foreign language in the presence of a resident that they cannot understand.

Communicating with your Supervisors and Co-Workers

Listening to Report and Completing Work Assignments

As a nursing assistant your supervisor will give you an oral report at the beginning of your shift. You will be updated with information on your residents that is important for you to know. Examples: reports could be about a resident who is depressed regarding a recent death in the family, a resident who needs to be ready for lunch out with a relative, a resident who is not to have food or fluids awaiting a medical test, or a resident who needs to be watched for any indications of pain. This type of information helps you meet the resident's needs. It is recommended that you carry a little note pad and pen to write down notes and reminders to yourself.

Your supervisor will at the beginning of the shift give you your work assignments. If you have any questions or concerns, seek clarification with your supervisor regarding the work assignment. Report back to the nurse any pertinent observations you make or inability to complete the assignment.

Resident Care Conferences

Care conferences are held periodically with representatives from various departments, the resident and their family present. You may be asked to attend. The purpose of the meeting is to identify current problems, set goals for resolution of the problems and develop approaches to meet the goals. All persons attending are encouraged to participate and share suggestions. As the nursing assistant, you may be the person who spends most time with the resident, so you may have some very important insights and ideas. This is your opportunity to make suggestions that may be incorporated into how care is provided! Through this meeting, the resident's care plan is updated and new directions may be developed.

OBRA requires that the resident be involved in the care planning process. Residents and their families are invited to attend the care conferences and can direct their care. The resident has the right to refuse proposed care. The care conferences provide a good opportunity for the resident and their family to communicate with the health care team and provide input into their own care.

The Medical Record

As a nursing assistant you will have the important responsibility of reading directions for care of the resident, providing care and recording the care provided. Recording the care provided is called **documentation**. There are many forms that are in the **medical record**. The ones the nursing assistant will be recording on are the resident care flow sheet and flow sheets that monitor specific issues.

The medical record is an important record of care that can be subpoenaed as evidence in a legal case. It therefore must be documented (recorded) accurately.

Resident Care

Resident care flow sheets are information sheets that give directions for care. They should be read carefully at the beginning of your shift so you can complete the assignment. After completion of the task, document that you have completed the task. Every resident has a resident care flow sheet or sheets. This is part of the medical record. All documentation must be carefully completed. As part of the permanent medical record, it can be used in legal cases. It therefore must be complete, accurate, and truthful.

There may additionally be specific flow sheets that monitor weight, vital signs, meal completion, or bowel and bladder retraining.

RESIDENT CARE FLOW SHEET

NURSING ORDER	HOUR	1	2	3	4	5	6	7	8	9	10	11	12	13	14	15	16	17	18	19	20	21	22	23	24	25	26	27	28	29	30	31
	THRU																															
PROVIDE INCONTINENCE PROTECTION: BRIEFS & PADS. CHANGE Q 2 HRS.	NOCS																															
	DAYS																															
	EVES																															
USE APPROPRIATE SEATING &/OR DEVICE(S) WHEN OUT OF BED TO DECREASE RISK FOR FALLS	NOCS																															
	DAYS																															
	EVES																															
ONE PERSON TRANSFER. SUPPORT ON RIGHT SIDE, TRANSFER TOWARD LEFT SIDE																																
OFFER ONE GLASS H$_2$O BETWEEN MEALS AND HS ENCOURAGE TO DRINK ALL FLUID ON TRAYS	DAYS																															
	EVES																															
SET UP SUPPLIES. CUE TO WASH HANDS & FACE. ASSIST AS NEEDED TO COMPLETE TASK. DOCUMENT Y=ABLE N=NOT ABLE	DAYS Y/N																															
	INITIAL																															
	EVEN.Y/N																															
	INITIAL																															
SET UP SUPPLIES. CUE TO DO OWN ORAL HYGIENE. ASSIST AS NEEDED TO COMPLETE TASK. DOC Y=ABLE N=NOT ABLE	DAYS Y/N																															
	INITIAL																															
	EVEN.Y/N																															
	INITIAL																															
ALLOW TIME TO FEED SELF. SUPERVISE WITH PROMPTING & VERBAL CUEING. ASSIST AS NEEDED TO COMPLETE TASK. DOC Y=ABLE N=NOT ABLE	DAYS Y/N																															
	INITIAL																															
	EVEN.Y/N																															
	INITIAL																															
IS HOH IN RIGHT EAR, SPEAK INTO LEFT EAR.																																

SIGNATURES _____

RESIDENT NAME _____   ROOM/BED _____   FACILITY _____

Resident Care Plans

Every resident has a **care plan** that identifies problems, develops goals and lists actions to achieve these goals. The multi-disciplinary team has input into the care plan. The following are examples of problems and other disciplines in addition to nursing who may be involved.

Problems pertaining to...	Input from...
impaired mobility	physical therapist
diabetes	dietitian podiatrist physician
depression	psychiatrist social worker activities director
inability to feed self and/or dress self	occupational therapist

The OBRA requirement is that all residents be assessed and re-evaluated at appropriate intervals regarding their physical, mental and psychosocial status. The care plan needs to be updated when new problems develop or previous problems resolve. Any actions that the nursing assistant needs to do will be passed on to you verbally and also listed on the flow sheet. The charge nurse will coordinate and communicate these changes.

Documentation on the Medical Record

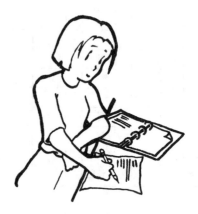

- ◆ All documentation must be done in pen.

- ◆ Do not erase, blacken or whiten out entries. If you make an error, draw one line through it. Write "error" above it and initial it.

- ◆ If you are not able to complete an assignment, write your initials with a circle around it and write out an explanation on the back of the sheet. Also verbally inform your charge nurse of not completing the assignment. Do not leave blanks.

- ◆ Be accurate, truthful and thorough in completing the medical record. Do not record opinions or judgements, just facts!

- ◆ Complete the record after completing the task you are documenting.

- ◆ Sign all documentation with your full name and title.

- ◆ Only chart for care that you provided.

Objective information is anything you can see, touch, smell or hear. This is tangible information with evidence. Examples: If you <u>see</u> a resident vomiting or if you <u>see</u> a resident fall, this is objective information.

Subjective information is information that you are told about and not able to observe directly. Examples: If a resident says he is nauseated or if a resident tells you that they fell earlier, this is subjective information.

Documentation should be objective. Comments the resident makes should be identified as such with quotation marks around their statement. Do not include your opinions or suspicions in written documentation.

Making observations

One of the very important skills a nursing assistant must have is making good observations regarding changes in the resident. Since it is the nursing assistant who is with the resident the most, the NA has the best opportunity to make observations. It is crucial that the NA realize what an important change is and in that instance to notify the supervisor. If you do not know the significance of the change it is best to check with the supervisor. Prompt reporting of any changes may help maintain the well being of the resident or even save his/her life.

Making good observations means using your senses of sight, hearing, touch and smell and being alert at all times to changes in the resident. You can use every opportunity you are with the resident to utilize your senses in the observation process. When you are giving a bath or shower you can observe the skin over the entire body. In particular, you are looking for reddened or irritated areas, beginning signs of a decubitus ulcer especially over bony prominences, sores, wounds, open areas, cuts, bruises, etc. You can also use this time to engage the resident in conversation and ask questions, from which you can learn about the resident's feelings and concerns. You can observe how the resident moves, their strength and coordination.

Carry a pad and pen with you while providing care so you can write down important observation. This will help you remember what you need to report to your charge nurse or what you need to document.

Visual observations

Skin

Bruising

Bluish area especially around lips and nailbeds due to lack of oxygen (cyanosis)

Breaks in skin

Signs of decubitus ulcer, especially over bony prominences such as coccyx, hips and heels

Edema (fluid retention in the tissues)

Wound drainage (observe color, consistency, amount)

Nasal / eye secretions (observe color, consistency, amount)

Cuts or bleeding

Respirations

Rapid, labored, irregular, or noisy

Any complaints of pain or difficulty breathing

Is the person coughing? Is the cough productive?

Unusual body alignment

One leg slightly shorter and rotating inward

Weakness

Is there new one-sided weakness, generalized weakness, or weakness on one side of the face?

Is safe movement affected?

Bowel movements and urine

Changes in frequency, color, amount

Incontinent

Unusual odor or appearance

Behavior change

Agitated, combative, withdrawn

Seizure activity

Eating and drinking

Usual amount

Difficulty chewing or swallowing

Food and/or fluids running out of one side of mouth

Participation in activities of daily living

Change in normal level of activity

Observations made by hearing

Resident's verbal expression of concerns, complaints, or suicidal thoughts

Change in speech, slurred speech, not being able to speak (aphasia) or speaking with difficulty

Confused speech

Noisy or congested breathing

Complaints of pain

Observations made by touch

Skin hot to touch or unusually cool to touch

Dry or rough skin

Pulse (rapid, slow or irregular)

Observations made by smell

Fruity breath

Unusually strong urine odor

Strong odors associated with poor personal hygiene

Odors pertaining to drainage or vomitus

Observations that should be reported immediately!

Changes in level of conciousness

Symptoms of myocardial infarction (heart attack) – crushing, squeezing, pain or pressure in the chest, nausea, dizziness, cyanosis, pain in one or both arms, back or jaw, dyspnea

Symtoms of cerebrovascular accident (stroke) – sudden weakness, numbness or paralysis of one side of the body, face, arm or leg, difficulty speaking, confusion, impaired vision, loss of balance, unconsciousness, loss of bowel control

A fall or injury

Bleeding

Complaints of pain

Abnormal vital signs

A newly discovered bruise, open or reddened skin area

Complaints of difficulty breathing or shortness of breath

Cyanosis around fingertips, nailbeds, and lips

Changes in mobility level

Behavioral changes such as combativeness, agitation, suicidal thoughts, being withdrawn, etc.

Vomiting

Refusing food or fluids

Observations regarding pain

Residents may suffer pain for a variety of reasons whether it is chronic pain perhaps due to arthritis, acute pain due to cancer, a fracture, surgery, or trauma. Many other conditions can result in pain. Pain also can be a very important indicator that something is wrong such as pain and discomfort related to a heart attack. It therefore is an important observation that needs to be made and reported to your supervisor immediately.

Residents may verbally tell you they are in pain but other residents may not be able to do so because of denial, or inability to communicate. Observe for the following signs and symptoms of pain.

- ◆ Crying or moaning, especially on movement or transfers
- ◆ Grimacing facial expressions
- ◆ Guarded positioning
- ◆ Behavior change for unknown reason
- ◆ Change in respirations, and holding breath
- ◆ Restlessness, irritability and/or fatigue

Report these signs and symptoms immediately to your supervisor. Pain management steps can then be implemented to bring relief to the resident.

Pain Management

Complaints of pain should never be ignored nor should anyone make judgments as to the validity or severity of pain a person is experiencing. Report the exact description the resident gives you. You play a crucial role in identifying pain so your supervisor can make a nursing assessment and help the resident achieve comfort.

Health care facilities have different ways to more objectively identify levels of pain. One method is to use a scale of 0 to 10 (0 indicating no pain, and 10 indicating worst pain possible). Other forms may show faces, ranging from a smiling face to a face with tears. Residents indicate the level of pain that they are experiencing. This is periodically documented and assessed by the RN or LPN. The RN or LPN may administer pain medication as ordered by the physician. Residents are carefully observed for their response to the pain medication with pain control being the objective. If the existing pain management plan is not effective, the RN will consult with the physician. There are also physicians who specialize in pain management who could be helpful. Helping a resident achieve comfort and a feeling of well being is an important part of nursing care.

Chapter 3 - Quiz Yourself

Circle the one correct answer

1. If you did not complete an assignment, what should you do on the flow sheet?

   a. Write in your initials, circle them and notify the charge nurse.
   b. Leave a blank.
   c. Tell the nurse about not being able to complete the task.

2. Smiles, frowns and gestures are examples of...

   a. Verbal communication
   b. Non-verbal communication

3. Aphasia means...

   a. Difficulty swallowing
   b. Confusion
   c. Difficulty speaking and/or understanding speech

4. When speaking to a resident in a wheelchair...

   a. Speak to them while standing.
   b. Speak to them while walking out of the room.
   c. Bend down to their level and speak while making eye contact.

5. Which of the following would make the resident feel that you are really listening to them?

   a. Standing with your arms crossed.
   b. Listening to them while you have your hand on the door knob.
   c. Frequently interrupting them.
   d. Making eye contact. Patiently allowing residents to express themselves and seeking clarification when needed.

Give an example of...

6. physical block to communication

_____

7. mental block to communication

_____

8. emotional block to communication

_____

Describe 2 observations you can make regarding...

9. skin

_____

10. respirations

_____

11. behavioral changes

_____

12. eating or drinking

_____

Answer these questions

13. Name 2 observations you should report immediately to the charge nurse.

_____

_____

14. Mrs. J. has aphasia after a recent stroke and is very difficult to understand. She is trying very hard to make herself understood and is getting increasingly frustrated. Describe what you can do to make communication easier.

_____

_____

15. Mr. S. has Alzheimer disease and cannot seem to understand what you are saying. Describe what you can do to make communication more effective.

_____

_____

True or False

16. _____ It is alright to use a pencil when writing on the medical record.

17. _____ The medical record is a legal record and can be subpoenaed in case of a lawsuit.

18. _____ If a resident is hard of hearing, you should shout.

19. _____ If you and your co-worker speak a foreign language that the resident does not understand, it is acceptable to speak it while taking care of the resident.

20. _____ If the resident says something that does not make sense, argue with them until you convince them that they are wrong.

Chapter 4
Medical Terminology and Abbreviations

Learning Objectives

1. Understand all medical terminology words listed in this chapter.

2. Know all abbreviations listed in this chapter.

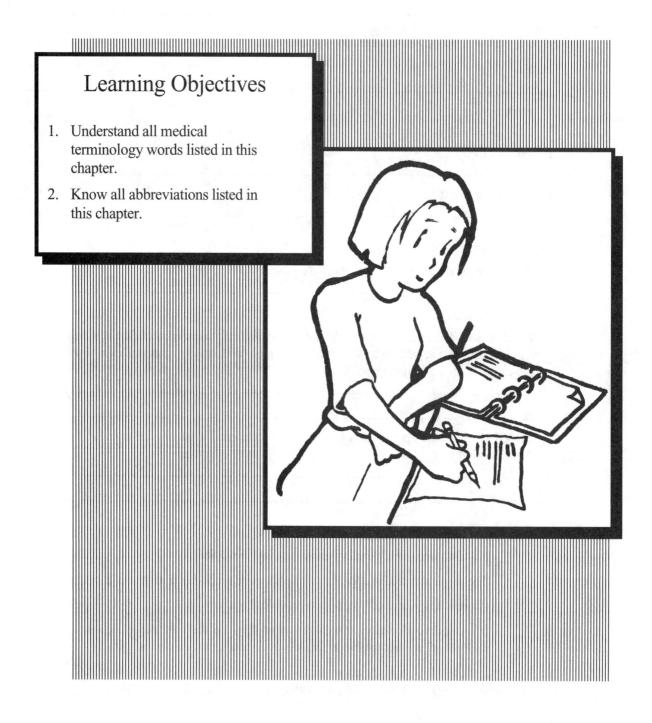

Medical terminology is based on the Latin and Greek languages. Learning medical terminology is like learning a new language. It is something you can start now and continue to build upon during your professional life. Buy yourself a pocket medical dictionary and use it when you come across a term you don't know.

In breaking down or trying to figure out a medical term, you can consider the following three parts...

- ◆ **word root** - the main part of the word
- ◆ **prefix** - a part added in front of the root word that adds meaning.
- ◆ **suffix** - a part added to the end of the root word that adds meaning.

The following are common **root words** & their meanings...

arthro - joint	**encephalo** - brain	**ped** - child
carcino - cancer	**gastro** - stomach	**plegia** - paralysis
cardia or cardio - heart	**hemo or hemato** - blood	**pnea** - breathing
cephalo - head	**hepa or hepato** - liver	**recto** - rectum
cerebro - cerebrum (brain)	**nephro** - kidney	**rhino** - nose
colo - colon	**neuro** - nerve	**sepsis** - infection
cysto - bladder	**osteo** - bone	**thrombo** - clot
derma - skin	**path** - disease	

The following are common **prefixes** that are added in **front** of root words and their meanings...

a or an - without, lack of	**hetero** - different	**myo** - muscle
auto - self	**homo** - same	**poly** - many
bi - two	**hydro** - water	**post** - after
brady - slow	**hyper** - above	**pseudo** - false
colo - colon	**hypo** - below	**quad** - four
contra - against	**micro** - small	**tachy** - fast
dys - painful	**mid** - middle	
hemi - half	**mono** - one	

The following are common **suffixes** that come at the **end** of the word and their meanings...

algia - pain   **ize** - remove   **path** - disease

cide - kill   **lysis** - destruction   **phasia** - speech

cyte - cell   **megaly** - enlargement   **plasty** - surgical repair

ectomy - removal of   **ology** - study of   **stenosis** - narrow

graph - record or picture   **oscopy** - look into   **uria** - urine

itis - inflammation   **ostomy** - surgical opening

Putting Words Together

A prefix is a word element placed at the beginning of a word used to change the meaning of a word. What do the following prefixes mean and what does the entire word mean?

	Prefix meaning	**Word meaning**
a- as in asepsis	without	without infection
brady- as in bradycardia		
hemi- as in hemiplegia		
micro- as in microorganism		
tachy- as in tachycardia		
dys- as in dyspnea		
quad- as in quadriplegia		

A root word contains the basic meaning of the word. What do the following mean?

	Root word meaning	**Word meaning**
cardio- as in cardiovascular	heart	heart and blood vessels
hepa- as in hepatitis		
gastro- as in gastritis		
osteo- as in osteoporosis		
cerebro- as in cerebrovascular accident		
colo- as in colitis		

A suffix is a word element placed at the end of a word to change the meaning. What do the following mean?

	Suffix meaning	Word meaning
ectomy- as in tonsillectomy	removal of	removal of tonsils
itis- as in appendicitis		
ology- as in pathology		
plegia- as in hemiplegia		
oscopy- as in colonoscopy		
ostomy- as in colostomy		
plasty- as in rhinoplasty		

Abbreviations

@	at	BM	bowel movement
$\bar{a}$	before	BP	blood pressure
abd	abdomen	BR	bed rest
ac	before meals	BRP	bathroom privileges (a person is allowed to get out of bed and ambulate to the bathroom on his/her own)
ad lib	as desired		
ADL's	activities of daily living	C	Celsius, also Centigrade
AIDS	acquired immune-deficiency syndrome	$\bar{c}$	with
		c/o	complains of
AKA	above knee amputation	Ca	cancer
am	morning	cardio	heart
amb	ambulate (walking)	cath.	catheter
amt	amount	CBR	complete bed rest
ax	axillary (underarm)	cc	cubic centimeter
B&B	bowel and bladder	CCU	cardiac care unit
BID	twice a day, 2 x day	cerebro	brain
BKA	below knee amputation		

CHF	congestive heart failure	HIV	human immunodeficiency virus
COPD	chronic obstructive pulmonary disease	HOB	head of bed
CPR	cardio pulmonary resuscitation	HOH	hard of hearing
CVA	cerebrovascular accident (stroke)	HS	hour of sleep, bedtime
DC	discontinue	ht	height
DNR	do not resuscitate	Hx	history of
DOE	dyspnea on exertion	hyper	above
Dx	diagnosis	hypo	below
ETOH	alcohol	I+0	intake & output
F	Fahrenheit	ICU	intensive care unit
F/u	follow up	in	inches
FBS	fasting blood sugar	inc.	incontinent
ft	feet	IV	intravenous (into blood vessel)
FWB	full weight bearing	L	left or liter
fx	fracture	LE	lower extremity
gal	gallon		RLE right lower extremity (leg)
GI	gastro intestinal		LLE left lower extremity (leg)
gt	one drop	lb	pound
GT	gastrostomy tube	LOC	level of consciousness
GTT	glucose tolerance test	LPN	licensed practical nurse
gtt	two drops	MD	medical doctor
GU	genito-urinary	MI	myocardial infarction (heart attack)
gyn	gynecology	min	minute
H	hour	ml	milliliter
H_2O	water	MRSA	methicillin resistant staphylococcus aureus
HBV	hepatitis B virus	MS	multiple sclerosis
hemi	half	NA	nursing assistant
hepat	liver	NAC	nursing assistant certified

NAR	nursing assistant registered		RN	registered nurse
naso	nose		R/O	rule out
NG	nasogastric		ROM	range of motion
NKA	no known allergies			PROM-passive range of motion
noc.	at night			AROM-active range of motion
NPO	nothing per os (nothing by mouth)		Rx	prescription, treatment
O_2	oxygen		$\overline{s}$	without
OBRA	Omnibus Budget Reconciliation Act		SBA	stand by assistance
OOB	out of bed		SOB	short of breath
OR	operating room		spec.	specimen (sample)
os	opening or mouth		stat	immediately
OT	occupational therapy		STD	sexually transmitted disease
oz	ounce		T	temperature
$\overline{p}$	post, after		TB	tuberculosis
pc	after meals		tbsp	tablespoon
per	by, through		TID	three times a day, 3 x day
pm	evening		TPR	temperature, pulse, respiration
po	per os, by mouth		tx	treatment
post op	after surgery		UA	urinalysis
PPE	personal protective equipment		UE	upper extremity
PRN	as necessary			RUE-right upper extremity (arm)
pt	patient			LUE-left upper extremity (arm)
PT	physical therapy		URI	upper respiratory infection
Q	every		UTI	urinary tract infection
Q2h	every 2 hours		VRE	vancomycin resistant enterococcus
QH	every hour		VS	vital signs (temperature, pulse, respirations & blood pressure)
QID	4 times a day		w/c	wheelchair
R	right, rectal, or respirations		WT	weight

a

abdomen- area between chest and pelvis.

abduction- moving arm or leg away from the body.

abuse- hurting a person by treating them badly.

acquired immunodeficiency syndrome- a disease that destroys the immune system leading to death caused by HIV.

active range of motion (AROM)- a person can move joints fully on their own.

activities of daily living- activities that people do every day such as bathing, dressing, feeding, toileting, etc.

adduction- moving arm or leg to the center of the body.

advanced directive- a person signs a document that makes arrangements for future health care decisions in the event that the person may not be able to make decisions. Two different types are "Healthcare Durable Power of Attorney" and the "Living Will".

agitated- anxious, nervous.

alcohol prep- small pad soaked with disinfectant alcohol used to clean skin.

alignment- keeping a straight line.

Alzheimer disease- terminal disease resulting in dementia.

ambulatory- able to walk.

amputation- removal of all or part of arm, leg, finger, etc.

anal- pertaining to the anus.

angina- chest pain because heart is deprived of oxygen.

antibiotics- drugs designed to kill bacteria that cause disease.

antibody- is part of the immune system to identify and fight pathogens such as viruses and bacteria.

antiseptic- cleaning that prevents growth of bacteria.

anus- opening in the body from which feces is excreted.

aorta- large blood vessel carrying blood and oxygen away from heart.

aphasia- unable to speak or understand speech.

apical pulse- obtaining a pulse by listening through a stethoscope placed over the heart.

arteriosclerosis- thickening and hardening of wall of arteries frequently associated with aging.

artery- blood vessel that carries blood away from the heart.

arthritis- can refer to joint pain or joint disease. There are more than 100 different types of arthritis and related conditions.

artificial- not real.

asepsis- to be free of disease causing microorganisms

aspirate- inhaling food or fluid into lungs.

atherosclerosis- artery disease due to deposits of fatty substances on inner artery walls.

atrophy- shriveling, wasting away, weakening.

axillary- underarm area.

b

bacteria- is a single-celled microorganism. Some bacteria is beneficial to good health, especially related to digestion. Other bacteria are behind serious illnesses like strep throat, food poisoning and pneumonia.

battery- touching another person without their permission.

bedpan- pan that the resident uses for a bowel movement or passing urine.

bedridden- unable to get out of bed.

bladder- muscular sac for storage of urine.

blood pressure- force of blood inside the artery wall. This pressure is measured at two points; when the heart contracts and when it relaxes.

body language- non verbal communication such as posture, grimacing, facial expressions, smiles.

body mechanics- the way we stand and move our body.

bony prominence- place where bones are close to surface of skin.

bowel movements- to pass stool as final process of digestion.

brachial pulse- pulse on the inside of the elbow, above the bend in the elbow.

c

calibrated- measured.

cancer- cells that grow out of control spreading and destroying healthy cells.

cane- walking stick used for balance or to support weight.

carcinoma- cancers that begin in the cells that make up skin or tissue lining organs These cancers can include skin cancer, prostate, colon, breast, lung, liver or kidney cancer.

cardiac arrest- lack of heart beat.

cardiac- pertaining to the heart.

cardiopulmonary resuscitation (CPR)- done when the patient has no heart beat and respirations. Circulation is maintained by doing chest compressions, and doing mouth to mouth respiration to prevent death of brain cells.

carotid pulse- pulse on either side of neck.

cataract- clouding of the lens of the eye.

catheter- tube inserted into body opening.

catheterization- inserting a catheter.

cell-basic unit of living matter, the smallest form of life.

central nervous system- brain and spine

cerebral- pertaining to the brain.

cerebrovascular accident (CVA)-stroke, interruption of blood and oxygen to part of the brain. Caused by a blockage in a blood vessel or a ruptured blood vessel.

circulation- movement of blood through the blood vessels and throughout the body.

clean catch urine specimen- obtaining urine sample during middle of urinary stream

clinitest- measurement of glucose in urine.

coccyx- bone at the base of the spine.

colon- large bowel or intestines

colostomy- surgical opening into the colon.

coma- unconscious state

combative- fighting, striking out or hitting

commode- a movable chair used for toileting with a bed pan in it

communicable- disease that can be passed on

confidentiality- keeping information about resident private.

congested- filled with fluid.

constipation- infrequent passing of hard stool

contagious- spread of infection or disease from person to person

contaminate- to make dirty or contaminate with microorganisms

contract- become smaller

contracture- muscle that becomes shortened due to lack of use

cueing- to remind, prompt or talk someone through an activity.

cyanosis- blue or gray color that appears on nail bed, or lips due to lack of oxygen in the blood

d

dangling position- resident sits with their legs over the side of the bed.

decubitus ulcer- breakdown of tissue, usually over bony prominences when circulation to the area is poor.

defecate- to have bowel movement, to pass stool.

dehydration- inadequate intake of fluids.

dementia- impaired mental and intellectual function.

dentures- artificial teeth.

depression- grief or sadness.

dermis- inner layer of skin.

diabetes mellitus- a chronic disease in which the pancreas does not produce enough insulin.

diagnosis- disease or condition a patient may have as identified by a physician.

diarrhea- loose, fluid discharge from the bowel.

diastolic blood pressure- the pressure in the blood vessels when the heart relaxes between contractions. This appears as the bottom number of the blood pressure.

digestion- mechanical and chemical breakdown of food that turns food into useable energy source for the body.

dirty- object or area contaminated by harmful micro-organisms.

disability- loss of ability

disinfection- destroying most disease-causing organisms.

disoriented- confused as to time, date, place and environment.

draw sheet- a small bed sheet placed crosswise over the middle of the bottom sheet covering the area between the person's upper back and thighs. Caregivers standing on each side of the bed can then move the patient up in bed by lifting the draw sheet.

dyspnea- difficult, painful, or labored breathing.

e

edema- fluid retention resulting in swelling.

elimination- to expel, to excrete waste products.

embolus- a blood clot that travels from one point and lodges in another blood vessel causing a blockage.

emergency medical service (EMT)- police, fire or first aid paramedic response to emergencies.

emesis basin- small kidney shaped basin into which resident will vomit or spit.

emesis- vomitus

endocrine system- glands that produce hormones that regulate growth, development, metabolism, sleep, sexual function, reproduction, and mood. The eight major glands include the pituitary gland, pancreas, ovaries, testes, thyroid, etc.

enema- introduction of fluid into rectum and colon to relieve constipation.

epiglottis- trap door that leads to lungs that prevents food from entering airway.

esophagus- tube for passage of food, from throat into stomach.

exhaling-breathing air out.

expectorate- to spit.

extension- to straighten an arm or leg.

extremities- arms and legs.

f

false imprisonment- restricting a persons movements when the resident poses no danger to himself or others.

fecal- pertaining to feces

feces- stool, bowel movement, solid waste material excreted from rectum.

fever elevated temperature

flatus- gas expelled from digestive tract

flexion- bending motion

flow sheet- a form used to document resident information, such as recording ADL's or vital signs

Foley catheter- a tube (catheter) inserted into the bladder to drain urine

foot drop- a contracture of the heel cord resulting in shortening of the muscles in the calf of the leg

force fluids- encouraging resident to take in extra fluids as ordered by the physician.

Fowler's position- sitting up in bed position with head of the bed rolled up 45°.

fracture- broken bone

fracture pan- bedpan with a lower flat end helpful to residents who cannot move easily.

g

gait belt- belt helpful in transferring residents

gait- walk or stride

gangrene- death of tissue due to either obstructed circulation or bacterial infection.

gastrointestinal system- (G.I.) stomach and intestinal system; digestive tract

geriatric- pertaining to the aged

geri-chair- a chair with wheels and a tray that locks in place

gesture- using your hands as communication

glaucoma- increased pressure in the eyeball.

graduate- measuring cup marked along the side (calibrated) for measurement of fluids.

h

hand roll- roll placed in the hand to prevent hand contraction

hazard- danger

health care directives- written instructions a person may leave as to what they would like done regarding end of life issues in the event they are not able to make these decisions later.

hemiparesis- loss of sensation on one side of the body.

hemiplegia- paralysis of one side of the body

hemorrhage- excessive blood loss

hemorrhoid- enlarged vein in rectum that causes pain and bleeding

hepatitis- inflammation of the liver

HIV- human immunodeficiency virus

homeostasis- balance of all body functions within normal limits.

hormones- substances secreted by the endocrine glands

human immunodeficiency virus (HIV) - the virus that causes AIDS, resulting in destruction of the immune system

hydration- adequate fluids

hygiene- cleanliness

Heimlich maneuver- a technique used to dislodge an airway blockage

hyperglycemia- high blood sugar

hypertension- high blood pressure

hypoglycemia- low blood sugar

hypotension- abnormally low blood pressure

i

immobility- not able to move

immune system- a complex system made up of cells, organs, and tissues that work together to protect the body from disease.

immunization- injections or oral vaccines to prevent communicable diseases

impaction- very hard stool that does not move

incontinence- lack of control over urine or stool

indwelling catheter- a tube that is put into the bladder to drain urine

infection- invasion and multiplication of microorganisms into the body such as viruses and bacteria that are not normally present.

inflammation- a localized reaction in the body with redness, swelling, heat, and pain in response to injury or infection.

inhalation- to breathe in

intake and output (I&O) - amount of fluid taken in and put out

inspiration- drawing in air

insulin- hormone produced by the pancreas which breaks down sugars and starches

integument- skin

intravenous- means "within a vein". It refers to giving medications or fluids through a needle or tube into a vein.

isolation- separation of infectious from non-infectious

j

joint- part of body where two bones come together

k

kidney- 2 organs in the upper back portion of the abdomen that remove waste products from the bloodstream and excrete them as urine

l

lateral- to the side of the body

laxatives- medication that makes it easier for a resident to pass a bowel movement

ligament- strong strands of tissue that connect bones together.

logroll- turning the resident onto the side, keeping the resident's head and back in a straight line

m

malignant- a tumor that spreads and is cancerous

medical asepsis- techniques and procedures to decrease the spread of pathogens.

metastasis- spread of cancer throughout the body

microorganism- a living thing so small that cannot be seen by a naked eye. It requires a microscope to be seen.

midstream- obtaining a urine sample after the resident starts the stream

mucus membrane- lining inside certain passages of the body such as nose, lungs, rectum, genital area

myocardial infarction (MI)- heart attack

n

nasal- pertaining to the nose

nasogastric tube (NG tube)- A tube going from the nose to the stomach used to feed the resident.

nausea- a feeling that you want to vomit

negligence- failure to give care or use precautions which can result in harm or injury to the resident

nephron- basic filtering unit of the kidney

nervous system- the brain spinal cord, and nerves that control and regulate activities and functions of the body.

non-ambulatory- unable to walk

nonverbal- without words

nutrition- taking in and using food for proper function of the body

o

obese- overweight

Omnibus Budget Reconciliation Act (OBRA)- a federal law that focuses on care of the elderly in long term care facilities.

observation- noticing change regarding the resident by using your senses such as sight, hearing, touch, and smell.

Ombudsman- a person who investigates complaints on behalf of the resident

opportunistic disease- a disease that develops in a person who has a diminished immune system

oral- having to do with the mouth

organ- a part of the body that performs a certain function such as the heart, stomach, etc.

organism- living thing

osteoporosis- loss of calcium from the bones that results in bones fracturing very easily

ostomy- surgical opening into the body. An example is a surgical opening into the intestine so feces leaves the body through this opening instead of through the rectum.

output- amount of fluid a resident puts out.

oxygen- a gas element required for human life.

p

paralysis- inability to move a body part

paraplegia- paralysis of the lower limbs of the body

passive range of motion (PROM)- someone other than the patient moves the joint through its full range.

pathogens- disease causing microorganism

perineum- area between the anus and the scrotum or vulva.

peristalsis- churning like motion that pushes food through the digestive tract.

personal protective equipment (PPE)- masks, gowns, gloves, etc.

perspiration- sweat

physician- doctor

pneumonia- acute infection of the lungs

podiatrist- foot doctor

post mortem- after death

posterior- in the back

postoperative- after surgery

pressure ulcer- also known as decubitus ulcer or bedsore. a breakdown of tissue due to decreased circulation to the area

prominences (bony)- places on the body where bones come close to the surface, such as coccyx, heels, elbows.

pronation- a turning down motion

prone- lying on abdomen

prosthesis- artificial body part as in arm, hands, legs, feet, breasts, eyes.

protective or reverse isolation- isolation technique utilized to protect the resident from the pathogens in the environment.

psychological- having to do with thoughts, feelings and emotions.

Chapter 5

Safety and Emergency Procedures

Learning Objectives

1. Explain what the leading cause of injury to the resident is.

2. Explain why hip fractures are so dangerous to the elderly.

3. List at least 4 contributing causes of falls.

4. Explain when an accident / incident form would need to be filled out.

5. Describe 3 possible causes of fires.

6. Describe the order of action in case of fire.

7. Demonstrate CPR on a manikin.

8. Demonstrate abdominal thrusts on a manikin.

9. Describe at least 3 symptoms of a heart attack.

10. Describe how to know if a person has an airway obstruction.

11. Demonstrate use of AED on a manikin.

Terms to Know

fire extinguisher
abdominal thrusts
cardiopulmonary resuscitation (CPR)
heart attack (myocardial infarction)
automated external defibrillator (AED)

Safety is a major concern for the elderly. The most common accident is falling. 70% of accidents in nursing facilities are due to falls. As people age, falling can be a life-altering problem frequently resulting in the person losing their ability to live independently safely.

Twenty percent (20%) of nursing home admissions are due to falls. After a hip fracture at home, a person may be hospitalized and afterwards require nursing assistance while they recuperate. They may require ongoing assistance with ambulation, transferring and ADL's.

Other startling statistics are that 20% of people over the age of 65 will suffer a hip fracture, and of them, 30% will die within 6 months. A frequent complication after a hip fracture may be pneumonia, a very common killer of the elderly. Residents are particularly susceptible to pneumonia after a hip fracture because they are usually not as mobile as they were previously. The decreased level of mobility contributes to the amount of fluid built up in the lungs resulting in pneumonia. Therefore, falls can be deadly to both men and women and all precautions need to be taken to avoid them.

Why Do People Fall?

♦ Confusion and disorientation of the resident resulting in poor judgment, decreased awareness etc.

♦ Side effects of medications which might make them drowsy, confused or dizzy.

♦ Muscle weakness

♦ Paralysis due to stroke, spinal cord injury or head injury

♦ Right or left side neglect due to stroke

♦ Balance and coordination problem

♦ Slower reaction time associated with aging, causing resident to respond slowly to danger or emergencies

♦ Decreased vision or blindness. Vision aging changes include loss of depth perception, problems with vision adjusting to glare, and poor peripheral vision

♦ Decreased sense of touch

♦ Dizziness due to orthostatic hypotension (blood pressure drop on sudden position change)

♦ Osteoporosis (loss of calcium from the bones) resulting in bones becoming more brittle and susceptible to fractures. See more information on osteoporosis in Chapter 20 Common Health Problems.

♦ Chronic diseases affecting mobility and strength, such as Parkinson's disease, multiple sclerosis, etc.

♦ Pain

Environmental factors...

Unfamiliar surroundings or changed furniture placement

Spills on the floor

Clutter

Poor lighting

Use of extension cords or scatter rugs

Improper use of wheelchairs and canes

Improper footwear for resident

Slow staff response time to resident's call light

Failure to leave call light within reach of resident

Faulty equipment

Bed not returned to lowest position

Bed cranks not turned to out of way position

What can we do to improve resident safety?

♦ Always leave a signal light within reach of the resident. Teach the resident how to use it to summon help and be sure to respond promptly.

♦ Check on residents frequently according to the care plan and according to their needs.

♦ Leave the bed at its lowest position to make it easier for the resident to get in and out of bed and to reduce injury if a fall occurs.

♦ Make sure to lock brakes on wheelchairs, bed, commode, and stretchers.

♦ Make sure residents use only their own canes and crutches that are properly fitted to them.

♦ Insure that residents wear their hearing aids and put on clean eyeglasses if they wear them.

♦ Assist residents in putting on non-skid footwear. No floppy slippers or socks without soles.

♦ Assist residents with transfers as needed.

♦ Be sure to leave everything residents will need within easy reach.

How can we make the environment safer?

♦ Scatter rugs are not to be used

♦ Spills on the floor must be wiped up immediately by the first person who finds the spill.

♦ Tubs and showers must have non-skid mats or areas.

♦ Grab bars need to be available next to the toilet, shower and tub.

♦ Extension cords are not to be used and electrical cords are to be kept out of the way.

♦ All areas need to be will lit.

♦ Keep resident rooms hallways and all public areas clutter free.

♦ Hand rails in the hallways and on stairs are to be kept unobstructed.

What to do if a Person Falls

Our goal is to prevent falls from occurring but accidents unfortunately do happen. The gait belt provides a good place for support while ambulating people. Maintain a firm grip on the gait belt. If a person does start to fall, it is best to guide the fall and gently lower the person to the ground. You can injure yourself if you react impulsively while trying to break the fall.

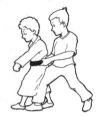

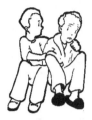

The charge nurse must deterimine that there are no injuries before the person can be moved. The move can be done by rolling the person onto a blanket. Position two caregivers on both sides. Caregivers kneel on one knee and grasp the blanket. On the count of three, lift the person and stand up. Move the person onto the bed.

Other types of accidents

Burns - can be caused by careless smoking or spills of hot fluids. Cigarettes, matches, and lighters should not be allowed in residents' rooms. The smoking policy should be diligently upheld because some residents may be confused and disoriented using poor judgment when smoking. Other residents may be drowsy and fall asleep while smoking; others may have poor motor control of their fingers resulting in a dropped cigarette. If a fire should occur in a health care facility, evacuation could be difficult because many residents have mobility problems.

Be careful regarding residents and hot fluids such as coffee, tea, etc, also check bath and shower temperatures.

Poisoning - Residents who are confused and/or have poor vision may eat or drink substances that are poisonous. Cleaning agents and disinfectants should be kept under lock and key at all times.

Choking, suffocation and asphyxiation - Interruption of respiration can quickly lead to death. Older residents who have swallowing disorders (dysphagia) such as after a stroke are more susceptible to choking. Improperly positioned residents and those who have improperly fitted dentures or no dentures or residents who do not properly chew are susceptible to choking. Residents who are weak and cannot independently change their position in bed may suffocate if they are put in a prone position (stomach laying position). Residents who are improperly restrained may strangle and suffocate if their position and restraint shifts. (See section on restraints)

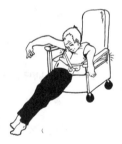

Accident / incident report

An incident is an unusual occurrence. If you, a visitor, or a resident is involved in an accident or incident, it must be immediately reported to the supervisor and an accident/incident report must be filled out. The report should be filled out as soon as possible so all details are fresh in people's minds and include witness observations. A report should be written even if there are no apparent injuries.

AED – automated external defibrillator is a machine that analyzes the hearts rhythm and if necessary, tells you to deliver a shock to a victim of sudden cardiac arrest. This shock is called defibrillation.

To Defibrillate – to deliver an electrical currency (shock) through the AED. This will interrupt ventricular fibrillation and return the heart to a normal healthy rhythm.

Cardiovascular - heart and blood vessel system (arteries, capillaries and veins)

Cardiac Arrest - when the heart beat and breathing stops suddenly. Caused by chaotic electrical impulses that result in an ineffective, irregular rhythm (ventricular fibrillation)

Myocardial Infarction - "heart attack". There is inadequate supply of oxygen to the heart muscle causing it to die. This can be due to a rhythm (contraction) problem or a blockage of a blood vessel that supplies the heart.

Angina Pectoris - Temporary pain or discomfort due to inadequate oxygen to the heart frequently brought on with physical exertion. It can radiate to the shoulders, arm, neck, jaw or back and last 2-15 minutes. It is relieved by rest and/or nitroglycerin.

Cardiopulmonary Resuscitation (CPR) Saves Lives!

Everyone in the general community needs to know CPR, but especially health care givers who may encounter situations when CPR is necessary. In the US every year, 1.5 million people have cardiac events (cardiac arrests, myocardial infarctions) and of them 500,000 die. The main objective of CPR is to provide oxygenated blood to the heart, brain and other vital organs until advanced medical help arrives.

85% of cardiac arrest victims have ventricular fibrillation (chaotic, ineffective rhythm), which necessitates an electrical shock called defibrillation. AED units are carried by Emergency Medical Service (EMS) and can alter this deadly rhythm and hopefully save the person's life. EMS help can be summoned by calling 911. Portable AED units are increasingly available in public locations. You will learn how to use AED as part of your CPR class so that you can use it if needed.

Time is a crucial factor in survival of the person who is in cardiac arrest. Brain damage can occur within 4 minutes after cardiac arrest and death can occur within 6-10 minutes. The person's best chance of survival is having someone do CPR which circulates blood throughout the body, thereby keeping vital organs alive until EMS arrives. EMS professionals will work on the scene to stabilize the person and transport to a cardiac care unit in a hospital.

Improving Survival Rate

A very important component is early recognition that the person indeed is having a life-threatening problem. This means realizing that the symptoms may require immediate professional assistance.

Symptoms of a Heart Attack

- ♦ A pressure in the chest. It is not a sharp pain but a crushing pressure and sensation in the chest. People also describe this as a tightness, achiness, or heaviness.

- ♦ Pain that radiates up into the jaw, neck and shoulders, one or both arms and back.

- ♦ shortness of breath

- ♦ nausea

- ♦ sweaty, clammy, diaphoretic feeling

- ♦ feeling weak

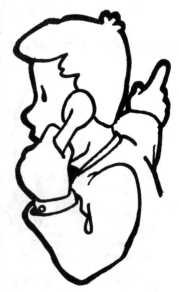

Not all symptoms will appear in all heart attack victims. If these symptoms last more than 2 minutes, seek help. The person should sit or lie down. A very common reaction however of this person is denial of the possibility that this may be serious and that they need to call 911. People may say or think things like "I'm too young," "I'm too healthy to have this happen," " I don't want to bother anyone". "What will my neighbors think when the AID unit arrives? Denial can prevent a person from seeking the help they need.

The sooner a person seeks professional help, the better their chance of survival. The longer they wait the greater the risk they will go into cardiac arrest and not be able to summon help. Current statistics indicate that 50% of people who had cardiac events arrived at the hospital by private transport, either driving themselves or having someone drive them. These people should have called 911 instead.

If a person does go into full cardiac arrest their chances of surviving it are drastically improved if someone promptly calls 911, initiates CPR and defibrillation occurs quickly. Recent studies indicate that if resuscitation occurs within one minute, the success rate may be 75%, if it occurs eight minutes later, the success rate may be only 6%. Chances of success are reduced 7-10% for each minute of delay. 77% of cardiac arrests occur in the home. The more people that know CPR and can start this life-saving technique before advanced medical help arrives, the better.

The specific steps of CPR and practice will be provided to you when you take a CPR class. The American Heart Association and the American Red Cross offer CPR classes. All health care workers need to be current in their CPR skills. Never practice on a person. This can be very dangerous to a conscious person.

The specifics for child and infant CPR are different. It is recommended that everyone also be current in these skills by taking an infant and child CPR class.

Health Care Provider CPR and Use of AED

1. Check for responsiveness of the victim. Tap the person on the shoulder and ask "Are you ok?". A person who is unresponsive is a person who does not move, makes no sounds, is not breathing, or is not breathing normally. (Gasps do not qualify as normal breathing).

2. If the person is unresponsive, activate the Emergency Response System (EMS) and get the AED. Send someone else to get the AED if possible.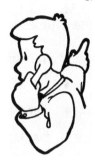

3. Check the carotid pulse for no more than 10 seconds.

4. If no pulse, start cycles of 30 compressions and 2 breaths. Chest compressions are done over the lower half of the sternum which compresses the heart. This in turn circulates blood and oxygen to the heart, brain, and other organs.

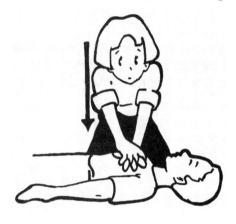

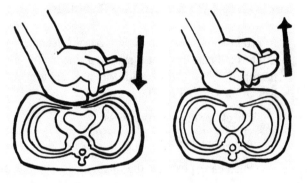

Push hard, push fast!
Compress the chest 2 inches, at a rate of 100 compressions per minute.
Allow the chest to completely recoil after each compression.

The person should be on a hard surface such as on the floor. When doing compressions, kneel over the person and keep your elbows straight.

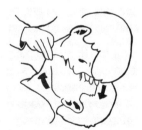

Open the airway by doing a head tilt, chin lift. Pinch the nostrils, put your mouth over the persons mouth and give a breath. Each breath should last over one second and result in the chest rising.

"If you are working in a health care facility you can use a bag mask to deliver breaths to the person. You will be taught how to do this in your CPR class".

5. Continue cycles of 30 compressions and 2 breaths until the AED or EMS arrives. If the rhythm is determined to be shockable give one shock and follow AED instructions. If the rhythm is determined to be not shockable, resume CPR immediately. Check for rhythm every two minutes and follow AED instructions. Continue until EMS arrives.

AED/Defibrillation

AED units have become much more "user-friendly". You will learn to use the AED in your CPR class. If an AED is available, use it! They are becoming increasingly available in health care facilities and public areas such as shopping malls, airports, on airplanes, in office buildings, etc.. If no AED unit is available, EMS will arrive with an AED unit and hopefully convert the person to an effective cardiac rhythm.

Once CPR starts, you should only stop if any of the following occurs...

- ♦ you are too exhausted to continue

- ♦ someone else who knows CPR takes over

- ♦ you see a valid "Do Not Resuscitate" order

- ♦ victim regains consciousness, pulse, and breathing

Hands Only CPR for the Lay Rescuer

In order to increase the likelihood of bystanders doing CPR, Hands Only CPR is recommended. Studies indicate that if it is started immediately upon witnessed collapse and compressions are done hard and fast, it can be a life saver. The simpler technique may help people overcome panic and hesitation to do CPR. The steps are...

Check for unresponsiveness.

Activate EMS.

Push hard, push fast until help arrives. (no respirations given)

Maintaining Heart Health

Currently heart disease is the number one cause of death in the US. We are increasingly becoming aware that our lifestyle can affect cardiac health. Some factors that affect the health of our heart...

- ♦ **Smoking** - Cigarette smokers experience a 70% greater risk of death due to heart disease.

- ♦ **Hypertension** (BP 140/90 or above) - Controlling weight and, exercise and decreasing salt in the diet may lower BP. A physician may additionally prescribe medications.

- ♦ **Elevated Cholesterol and Triglycerides** - this is the main fat (lipid) component of atherosclerotic deposits which contribute to coronary artery disease. It lines the blood vessels to the heart, causing a blockage and depriving the heart muscle of oxygen. A desirable overall cholesterol reading is 200 or less with a good ratio of "good" cholesterol versus "bad" cholesterol. Some people have a genetic predisposition to elevated cholesterol. Many can control it through a diet lower in red meat, eggs and animal fats.

- ♦ Obesity

- ♦ Lack of regular physical exercise

- ♦ Emotional stress

A factor we cannot control is a family history of heart disease. If you have a parent who died of heart disease under the age of 60, you may be at added risk.

Partial Airway Obstruction

A partial airway obstruction occurs when an object, usually food, partially blocks the airway. The person would be coughing, making high-pitched sounds and possibly turning blue. The person is able to speak. Allow the person to continue coughing while sitting in an upright position and hopefully dislodge the object. Do not hit the person on their back since it can actually cause the object to lodge completely in the airway. Do not leave the person alone since the partial obstruction could become a complete obstruction and require immediate intervention.

Ill and elderly residents are susceptible to choking because their swallowing reflex can be impaired, they may have poor fitting dentures, and have general weakness. Choking is likely to occur at mealtime, especially with large, poorly chewed pieces of meat and while talking and laughing while eating. Foods that may be problematic and contribute to choking are grapes, popcorn, hard candy and hot dogs.

Complete Airway Obstruction

A complete airway obstruction is a life threatening situation that leads to cardiac arrest. The signs of a complete obstruction are an inability to cough, or speak. They are not able to speak and usually will clutch their throat. When a person appears to be choking, ask them if they are alright. This is to elicit a response from them. If they are not able to speak, this **is** a complete airway obstruction and immediate intervention is needed to save their life.

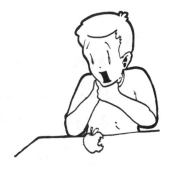

Clutching ones throat is considered a **universal sign of choking**.

Heimlich Maneuver

This is a procedure that is done to dislodge an airway obstruction. It causes the diaphragm to move upward, forcing air out of the lungs. This in turn can move the obstruction and force it out the mouth.

Procedure: Abdominal Thrusts (Heimlich maneuver) for the Conscious Victim

1. Stand behind the person. Place your hands around the mid section of the person slightly above the belly button.

2. Make a fist with your dominant hand with the thumb held inside the fist.

3. Place your fist with the thumb against the abdominal area, slightly above the naval.

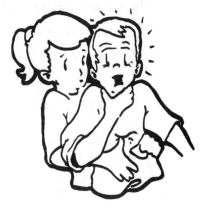

4. Grasp your fist with the other hand with your thumb toward the person.

5. Make one quick inward and upward thrust into the abdominal area.

6. Continue thrusts until the obstruction clears or the person becomes unconscious. If the person becomes unresponsive, lower them to the floor and continue with the following steps.

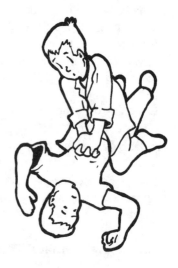

Procedure: Abdominal Thrusts for the Unconscious Victim

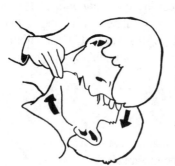

1. Activate emergency medical services by calling 911.

2. Place the person in a supine position. Open the airway by using the head tilt, chin lift maneuver.

3. If there is no breathing, give 2 ventilations. If the air did not enter, attempt 2 more ventilations.

4. If the air still does not enter the airway, kneel and straddle the person's thighs.

5. With your fingers pointing toward the person's chest, place the heel of one hand slightly above the naval. Place your other hand over the first hand.

6. Administer 5 inward and upward abdominal thrusts.

7. Open the person's mouth by doing a tongue-jaw lift maneuver. This is done by grasping the person's tongue and lifting the jaw forward with one hand.

8. While holding your index finger on the other hand in a hook position, sweep along the inside toward the base of the tongue.

9. Attempt to dislodge and remove any foreign objects, being careful not to push it deeper into the throat. Remove the object if possible.

10. Open the airway with the head-tilt, chin lift method.

11. Give one ventilation, repeat steps #4 to #9, and give one ventilation.

12. Repeat steps #4 through #11 until the airway clears.

Chapter 5 - Quiz Yourself

Safety - Circle the one correct answer

1. Falls in the elderly are dangerous because they can result in prolonged periods of immobility. This can lead to death due to...

   a. pneumonia
   b. bronchitis
   c. decubitus ulcer
   d. emphysema

2. An accident report should be filled out...

   a. immediately after the accident
   b. at the end of the shift
   c. at the end of the week

3. Which of the following residents are susceptible to choking?

   a. someone with dysphagia after a stroke
   b. a person who is not positioned properly in an upright position
   c. a resident without teeth or dentures
   d. all of the above

True or False

4. _____ The number one type of accident in a nursing home is a fall.

5. _____ Smoking is allowed in a room where oxygen is in use.

6. _____ In case of a fire, all residents in immediate danger should be evacuated first.

7. _____ ABC fire extinguishers can safely be used for all types of fires.

8. _____ When residents fall to the floor, assist them to their bed before notifying the charge nurse.

Fill in the answer

9. Name 3 environmental factors that can contribute to falls.

   _____

   _____

   _____

10. Name 3 medical conditions that may increase the risk of falling.

    _____

    _____

    _____

11. Describe the type of footwear a resident should have when standing, transferring, or ambulating.

    _____

Circle the one correct answer

12. CPR stands for...

    a. cerebropulmonary regurgitation
    b. cardiopulmonary resuscitation
    c. cerebro pulse release

13. The carotid pulse is at...

    a. the neck
    b. the wrist
    c. the groin
    d. the elbow

14. Myocardial infarction is another name for...

    a. stroke
    b. fainting
    c. heart attack

15. When doing CPR, you should do...

    a. 30 chest compressions and 2 breaths
    b. 10 chest compressions and 5 breaths
    c. 12 breaths and 6 compressions
    d. 10 breaths and 5 compressions

16. If a person has no heart beat and no respirations, they can start to have brain damage in...

    a. 1 minute
    b. 2 minutes
    c. 30 minutes
    d. 4 minutes

Fill in the answer

17. List 4 signs of a possible heart attack.

    _____   _____

    _____   _____

18. Why is it important to open the airway during CPR?

    _____

19. List 2 signs of a complete airway obstruction.

    _____   _____

20. If a resident is coughing and choking on food, what should you do?

    _____

Chapter 6
Restraints

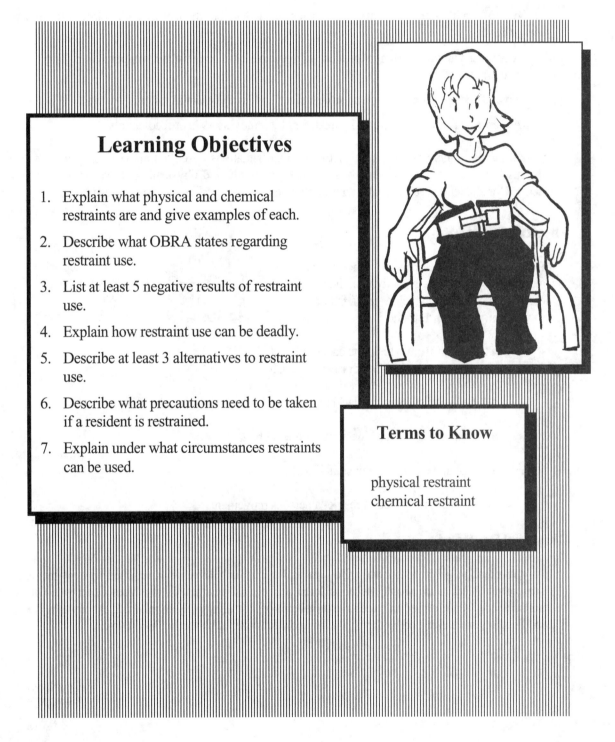

Learning Objectives

1. Explain what physical and chemical restraints are and give examples of each.

2. Describe what OBRA states regarding restraint use.

3. List at least 5 negative results of restraint use.

4. Explain how restraint use can be deadly.

5. Describe at least 3 alternatives to restraint use.

6. Describe what precautions need to be taken if a resident is restrained.

7. Explain under what circumstances restraints can be used.

Terms to Know

physical restraint
chemical restraint

You will encounter situations where maintaining safety will be challenging. The following represent just a few of these instances:

A person with dementia is at risk of wandering away from the facility with potential for injury or death.

A confused and/or weak person attempts to get out of a bed or chair without help risking a fall or injury.

An agitated or combative person strikes out at staff with potential for injury.

A confused person interferes with treatment by removing IV's or feeding tube.

Previously restraints were used freely to deal with situations described above. Today we realize that use of restraints can be devastating both emotionally and physically and can even result in death. Our challenge is to help maintain safety without having to resort to use of restraints.

Physical Restraints

Physical restraints include any method or equipment attached or adjacent to the body, that the individual cannot remove easily which restricts freedom of movement. Physical restraints include ...

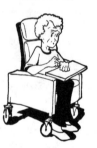

> A geri chair has a tray that locks in place making it a restraint.

♦ A chair from which one cannot get out of such as a Geri-chair or recliner chair.

♦ Belts, wrist restraints, jacket restraints, vest restraints, ties, hand mitts, etc.

♦ Bed rails that keep a person confined in bed.

♦ Holding a person against their will.

♦ A "bear hug" used to restrict a persons movement.

Chemical Restraints

Any medication given to control mood, mental status or behavior not required to treat medical symptoms. Medication would be considered a chemical restraint if it is prescribed when it is unnecessary, is prescribed in excessive doses and/or is inadequately monitored. As always, these medications are prescribed by the physician and administered by the licensed nurse.

OBRA Law and Restraints

OBRA law requires that restraints only be used when all appropriate alternatives have been used and they have been unsuccessful.

OBRA law states "the resident has the right to be free and the facility must ensure freedom from any restraint imposed or psychoactive drug administered for purposes of discipline or convenience, and not required to treat the resident's medical symptoms."

OBRA requires resident assessment and care planning in order "to attain and maintain the highest physical, mental and psychosocial well-being of each resident."

OBRA requires that care be provided in an environment that will promote maintenance or enhancement of the quality of life of each resident. The person must be informed of the reason for restraint use and that it is part of the plan of care. The physician or nurse will obtain consent. If the person is not able to give consent his/her legal representative will be contacted.

Our attitudes toward restraints today

Most health care facilities are restraint free facilities or at least working toward that goal. Due to the numerous negative results of restraint use, we need to work toward reducing or eliminating restraint use. Careful assessment can help identify alternative measures to prevent falls and injuries and maintain resident safety. Often the environment can be modified to reduce or eliminate restraint use. The least restrictive type of restraint should be used for the shortest amount of time.

What are the poor outcomes of restraint use?

Changes in body systems...

Sluggish blood in vessels

Cardiovascular stress

Incontinence

Weak muscles

Weakened bone structure

Pressure sores

Increased agitation

Depression

Decreased appetite

Increased pneumonia

Increased urinary infection

Changes in quality of life...

Reduced social contact

Withdrawal from surroundings

Less participation in activities

Loss of independent or assisted mobility

Loss of independent or assisted toileting

Loss of independent or assisted bathing/dressing

Decreased desire to eat

Increased problems with sleep pattern

Numerous studies on restraint use show that...

♦ the incidence of falls do not decrease when residents are restrained.

♦ agitation, resistance and other behavioral symptoms worsen when a resident is restrained.

The use of restraints results in tremendous loss of human dignity. Some comments residents have made as to how it makes them feel are...

> "I'm treated like a baby!"
> "Why am I being punished?"
> "Can't I be trusted at the age of 85?"
> "My feelings don't count"
> "I can't get up to go to the bathroom when I want"

Many other residents who are not able to verbally express their feelings show their distress non-verbally. They frequently tug and pull on their clothes or the restraint, yell for assistance, have anxious facial expressions and make repetitive motions. Withdrawn behavior is frequently seen, that is, the resident has down cast eyes, makes little eye contact and rarely initiates conversation.

Restraints Can Kill

Restraint use can turn deadly. Injury or death can occur in these ways...

♦ A resident in a Semi-Fowler's position and restrained in bed may slide down in bed causing the restraint to tighten around the chest and throat.

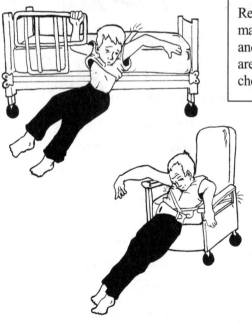

Residents restrained in bed with half rails up, may be able to get around to the end of the rail and dangle off the bed. Their weight, as they are suspended, may compress their throat or chest easily resulting in asphyxiation.

Residents restrained with a vest restraint in a bed with full side rails up may be able to climb over the rails. With the vest restraint still tied, they are left to dangle in mid-air, their throat, chest or abdomen compressed resulting in asphyxiation.

Residents restrained in a chair slip down, out of the seat with their buttocks on the floor. The vest restraint remains tied in place and tightens around the throat or chest resulting in asphyxiation.

Underlying principles for reducing restraint use

To decrease restraint use we need to evaluate and assess each case individually, develop a plan for each particular resident and as a health care team member, work toward this goal.

Resident assessment: in-depth assessment of a resident by interdisciplinary team including nurse, physician, dietician, social worker, pharmacologist, activities professional, and occupational, physical therapist, and speech therapist. Identification of strengths and weaknesses, including lifelong habits, daily routine, activities of daily living, mood, attitude, memory, communication, disease states, activities and medications. Assessment is continuous and ongoing throughout the stay.

Individualized care plan: plan based on strengths and deficits identified by assessment. Include resident and/or family or legal representative and nursing assistant in care planning conference. The care plan must meet *individualized* resident needs and change as resident needs change.

Teamwork: no one person or discipline has all the answers. Ideas may come from professional or non-professional direct care givers, indirect caregivers, volunteers, family and other residents.

Options For Action To Avoid Restraint Use

- ◆ Companionship and supervision including the use of volunteers, family, friends, etc.

- ◆ Physical and diversionary activity such as exercises, outdoor time, activities that resident would like to do, small jobs agreed to by the resident.

- ◆ Psychosocial interventions including meeting lifelong habits and patterns of daily activity.

- ◆ Environmental approaches: alarms, good lighting, reduced glare, mattress on floor to reduce falls, individualized seating.

- ◆ Meeting identified physical needs such as hunger, toileting, sleep, thirst and exercise according to individual routine rather than facility routine.

- ◆ Training staff to meet individualized needs.

- ◆ Staffing levels high enough to comply with the law which requires enough staff to meet residents' mental, physical and psychosocial needs. Use heavier staffing during peak periods of day.

Useful Devices to Replace Restraints

Ideally our goal is to prevent injuries while maintaining dignity and independence of the resident. There are devices that can now help toward this goal. The selection of the device useful for the resident requires careful assessment and evaluation. This is done by input from the multi-disciplinary team consisting of the physician, nursing dept., physical, occupational and restorative therapy, social services and most importantly the resident and their family.

Some helpful devices are...

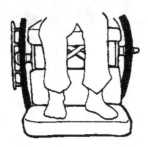

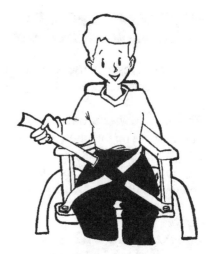

Height adjustable footrest extender - for good lower extremity positioning. This improves the base of support while sitting, improves body weight pressure distribution, and helps prevent foot drop. Resident's feet should never be allowed to dangle unsupported.

Resident release soft belt this is meant to eliminate poor wheelchair posture and sliding out of the chair. The residents can release the belts themselves. Some releases are even workable for the resident with poor hand dexterity.

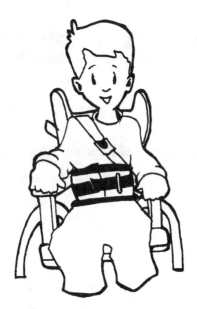

Total trunk support - ideal for residents with contractures that require support to maintain upright sitting position. Easy-open closures allow resident control over its use.

♦ **Wedge cushion** - helps the resident avoid sliding forward out of the chair by keeping their weight back in the chair. This keeps the knees higher than the buttocks.

♦ Various **alarms** that monitor the resident's movements.

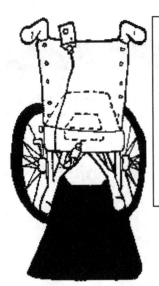

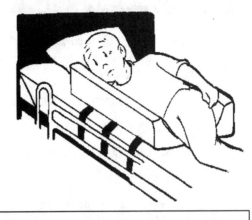

Alarm cushion - for wheelchair or geri-chairs. The pressure sensor in the cushion activates an alarm when the resident leaves the chair, alerting the staff to the situation.

Bed bolsters - these are bolsters that run half the length of the bed, reminding the resident not to get up and are an alternative to bed rail use.

Specific programs for reducing restraint use

The following programs help people to function more independently and improve their quality of life.

- Restorative care program including walking, bowel and bladder, independent eating, dressing, bathing programs.

- Wheelchair management program to assure that the correct size is used and that the resident is mobile by wheelchair.

- Individualized seating program for those residents who do not need wheels for mobility. Chairs should be tailored, the same way as wheelchairs, to individual needs.

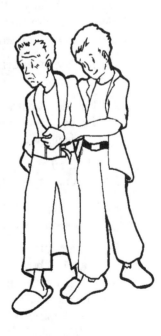

- Specialized programs for residents with dementia, designed to increased their quality of life during the day.

- Video visits - videotaped family visits when families live far away.

- Outdoor ambulation program every morning and afternoon in nice weather.

- Rehabilitation dining room to help residents increase mealtime skills and independence.

- Wandering program to allow safe wandering within an enclosed, supervised area, while preserving the rights of others.

- Preventive program for calming aggressive behaviors based on knowing the resident, preventing triggering of aggression and using protective intervention as a last resort.

Restraints can only be used if ordered by a physician or as ordered by the charge nurse in an emergency for a short time only. If a resident does require physical restraints the following **must be done every 2 hours**...

♦ Release restraint for at least 10 minutes.

♦ Toilet resident or check pad for dryness if appropriate

♦ If capable, stand and ambulate resident

♦ Offer fluids

♦ Check skin condition especially on buttocks and over bony prominences. Report any reddened or irritated areas to nurse immediately.

♦ Reposition

While restrained the resident needs to be checked every 30 minutes for safety. Tie restraints in such a way (half bow tie) as to release quickly in emergency. Do not tie to any bed part that can tighten the restraint when moved causing it to become dangerously tight for the resident.

Procedure: Applying a Vest (Posey) Restraint

Apply a restraint only if there is a physician's order for such and according to resident's care plan, and under the direction of the charge nurse. Follow the specific restraint manufacturer's recommendations for restraint application.

1. Explain to residents that you will be applying a restraint and answer any questions they may have.

2. Use the proper vest restraint size for the resident. Make sure it is not torn, cut, worn, or frayed. Apply the restraint over clothing, never directly over bare skin. In the female resident, make sure the straps are not directly over the breasts.

3. Adjust the straps so they are snug but not too tight. You should be able to insert two fingers between the restraint and the resident.

4. Make sure the resident is sitting comfortably and positioned well with any positioning devices necessary (wedge cushion, etc).

5. The restraint straps should be smooth and not twisted. Tie the straps using a quick release knot, half bow or slip knot, so the resident can be removed quickly in an emergency. Do not secure restraints to bed rails. If the resident is in a wheelchair tie it to the frame part of the wheelchair where the resident cannot reach to untie it. Put the vest ties through the slots at the sides of the seat, down and around the rear wheelchair legs. Check the restraint for appropriate tightness.

6. Check the resident every 30 minutes. Make sure they are still properly and safely positioned and that the restraint is not too tight. Check to make sure they have no circulation or breathing problems. Take care of any need the resident may have.

7. Every two hours, release the restraint, toilet them, ambulate if possible, offer fluids and reposition with restraint reapplied. Observe for any skin breakdown, redness, or irritation.

8. Place the call light within reach of the resident.

9. Leave fluids within reach of the resident.

10. Wash your hands.

11. Report any adverse change in behavior of the resident or problems with restraint use to the charge nurse.

Bed Rails

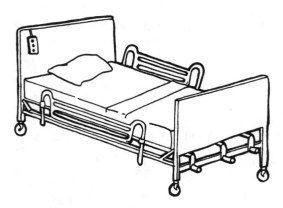

A bed rail or side rail is a barrier along the side of the bed. Bed rails can be raised or lowered and locked in place. Bed rails can run the entire length of the bed, be half or three quarter in length. The Resident's Care Flow Sheet will indicate whether a bed rail is to be used for the resident and if so, when. Bed rails are considered restraints, therefore they can only be used when ordered by the physician. However, there are additional circumstances under which they can be used...

♦ If the resident requests that bed rails be put up. In this case notify the charge nurse of this situation.

♦ Temporarily for safety or mobility purposes while providing direct care. An example would be putting up the bed rail while making an occupied bed. The bed rail would be put down as soon as the procedure is completed.

♦ During an emergency to insure safety of the resident. Notify the nurse of this situation immediately.

Bed rails can pose a danger to residents resulting in injury or death. Residents who are confused, or needing to go to the toilet desperately may climb over the rails resulting in a fall. This type of fall can result in a hip fracture or other injuries. Residents may potentially also become entrapped between the mattress and the bed rail. Check to make sure that the gap between the mattress and the bed rails or head board is not large enough to cause injury.

The following methods can help a resident stay safe without use of bed rails...

♦ Keeping a bed at its lowest position

♦ Using alarms that alert the staff when a resident attempts to get up

♦ Checking frequently with residents and assisting them as needed

♦ Placing pads on the floor near the bed to cushion possible falls

Chapter 6 - Quiz Yourself

Circle the correct answer

1. A medication used to control mood, mental status, and behavior is called a

    a. chemical restraint
    b. physical restraint

2. The restrained resident should be checked every...

    a. 30 minutes
    b. 2 ½ hours
    c. 1 hour
    d. 4 hours

3. The restrained resident needs to be released, ambulated, and toileted every...

    a. 30 minutes
    b. 1 hour
    c. 2 hours
    d. 6 hours

4. Which of the following are devices that are useful in replacing restraints?

    a. alarm cushion
    b. positioning cushion
    c. adjustable footrest extender
    d. all of the above

5. List 4 poor outcomes of restraint use.

    _____

    _____

    _____

    _____

True or False

6. _____ OBRA law allows use of restraints if it makes it easier for the nursing assistant.

7. _____ A geriatric chair with the tray locked in place is considered a restraint.

8. _____ A bed rail is not a restraint and can be put up anytime the nursing assistant feels it's necessary.

9. _____ Restraints can be deadly.

10. _____ It is acceptable to tie restraints to the bed rail.

Chapter 7

Body Mechanics, Positioning, and Ambulating Residents

Learning Objectives

1. State at least 4 reasons why proper positioning is important.

2. Demonstrate the following positions: supine, prone, Fowlers, semi-Fowlers, Trendelenburg, Sims.

3. Explain how the following devices are helpful: hand roll, foot boards, splints.

4. Explain how often residents should be repositioned and why this is important.

5. Define what contractures are and how they can be prevented.

6. Describe what can be done to prevent orthostatic hypotension.

7. Describe equipment that can aid ambulation and when they would be used.

8. Describe at least 5 rules of good body mechanics.

9. Explain when and why a gait belt should be used.

10. Explain when 2 or more caregivers are needed to transfer a resident.

11. Describe at least 3 assistive devices and when they need to be used.

Terms to Know

supine
prone
Fowlers
semi-Fowlers
foot board
foot drop
Trochanter roll
hand roll
contractures
atrophy
body alignment
Sims position
Trendelenburg position
ambulation
dangling
orthostatic hypotension
cane
crutches
walker
body mechanics
gait belt
Hoyer lift
slide board
trapeze bar
draw sheet
assistive device

These Are Four Steps You Must Take Before Starting Any Procedure

1. Wash your hands and use standard precautions including wearing gloves when appropriate.

2. Identify yourself to the resident and call them by name. Check their wrist band to establish identity.

3. Explain the procedure to the resident speaking clearly, slowly and directly while maintaining face to face contact whenever possible.

4. Provide privacy by closing doors, pulling privacy curtains, closing drapes or blinds.

End all procedures by doing the following...

1. Discard gloves if used.

2. Wash your hands.

3. Leave call signal within reach of resident.

4. Make sure that the resident is left in a safe and comfortable position.

Preventing Back Injuries

As a health care worker you are at special risk of back injury. The U.S. Department of Labor identifies nursing assistants as being at greater risk of workplace injuries as compared to other professions. Your job will involve lifting, transferring and moving residents often during the day. You will be transferring residents from bed to wheelchair, commode, toilet, chair, stretcher or gurney and back to bed again. You will be transferring residents who can partially assist or not able to assist at all.

When transferring human beings in the health care field as opposed to transferring objects in a warehouse or store, you have special considerations. If you came up to a 40 lb. box, you pretty much would know what to expect. When transferring a person however, the unexpected may happen at any time. A person may become faint, become a dead weight or become fearful or combative, incontinent or create a spill as they are being transferred. This element of the unexpected can result in an accident and back injury for you and the resident. Special care needs to be taken to prevent such injuries.

Understanding How Your Back Works

It is important to understand your back, how it works, what happens when an injury occurs and most importantly what to do to avoid injury.

Your spine is made up of vertebrae (bones) that float on discs (cartilage pads). The discs allow bending and flexibility of the back.

The spine has 3 parts...

- ◆ cervical (neck)

- ◆ thoracic (middle back)

- ◆ lumbar (lower back)

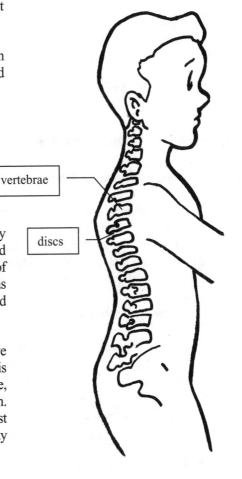

vertebrae

discs

The lumbar curve is especially vulnerable to injury because it balances and supports the upper body and because it can move and bend. Maintaining balance of these natural curves is important to prevent injury as well as keeping the supportive muscles of the back and abdomen toned.

When a person suffers a back injury they may have what is called a ruptured disc or herniated disc. That is where the disc may slip out of position or even rupture, pushing onto the surrounding nerves causing great pain. A person may feel very uncomfortable in most positions especially sitting or lying down and may experience pain radiating down a leg.

After an injury, physical therapy can be of help with a combination of rest, gentle stretching and strengthening exercises. Sometimes surgery is recommended. Of course prevention is most important in an effort to avoid this pain, discomfort and disruption of your enjoyment of life.

Things you can do to maintain good back health

- ◆ Maintain good posture to protect your spine. This means head held up, chin and stomach tucked in.

- ◆ Maintain strong flexible muscles of the abdomen and back and participate in a regular, conditioning exercise program such as walking, swimming etc.

- ◆ Learn and apply rules of good body mechanics in your daily life, both on the job and at home.

Body Mechanics

Good body mechanics means maintaining good body alignment (posture) when you are using and moving your body. Good alignment allows you to move your body with strength and effectiveness while avoiding muscle fatigue and strain and preventing injuries.

Poor body mechanics causes a disruption of the 3 natural curves (cervical, thoracic, and lumbar) due to improper body alignment.

Rules of Good Body Mechanics

1. Before Starting, Check Your Environment for Safety.

Make sure the area is well lit so you can see any spills on the floor, or objects that could be a hazard. Make sure the area is not cluttered. There should be no extension cords or scatter rugs. Make sure the wheelchair, commode chair and bed wheels are locked securely. The resident should have non-slippery footwear, never transferring in bare feet or stocking feet.

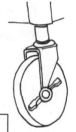

Make sure wheels are locked securely

2. Evaluate Your Load

Assess what or whom you will be lifting or moving. Before moving a resident make sure you find out from your charge nurse, from the care flow sheet or co-worker who is familiar with the resident, what the resident's limitations are. Do not rely on information from the resident unless you are absolutely certain that they are alert, oriented and that the information they will provide is accurate. You need to know...

- ◆ Can the resident bear weight?

- ◆ Is their strength equal on both sides?

- ◆ Can the resident hear and understand directions?

- ◆ Is this a one or two person transfer, or is a Mechanical lift required?

3. Get Close To Your Load

This can greatly minimize the load on your back. Avoid reaching over and get as close as you can to whatever you are lifting.

4. Stand With Your Feet 8-12 Inches Apart for A Wide Base of Support.

This will provide you stability and make you less vulnerable to falling.

5. Bend at the Knees

This utilizes your longest and strongest muscles, the thighs into the move. This relieves some stress on the shoulders, arms and back.

6. Keep Your Back Straight. Do Not Bend At the Waist!

Keep reminding yourself of this very important point until it comes naturally to you with each lift.

7. Move Your Torso (Area from Your Shoulders to Your Hips) As One Unit.

Don't twist your back when moving. Make sure your feet are pointing in the direction of the move.

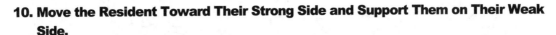
gait belt

8. Use A Gait Belt (Transfer Belt) When Moving A Resident.

This gives you a stable place to hold onto the resident. Do **not** have the resident put their arms around your neck.

9. When Possible Push, Pull Or Roll an Object to Minimize Risk to Your Back.

This decreases the risk of suffering a back injury.

10. Move the Resident Toward Their Strong Side and Support Them on Their Weak Side.

You must first of all know if the resident has a weaker side and plan the move accordingly. Place the chair you are transferring the resident to on their strong side. For a resident with one sided weakness or paralysis, stand and assist the resident on their affected side. If they are paralyzed on the right side, support them on their right side.

11. One Person Transfer Requires That The Resident Have At Least One Good Leg To Stand On. If They Do Not, It Will Require At Least a Two-Person Transfer, Or Transfer by a Hoyer Lift.

A "good" leg is one that is strong and can bear weight. It is not contractured, weak, paralyzed or missing (amputated).

12. Ask For Help If Necessary.

Better safe than sorry. Falls can lead to injuries. Approach all transfers with caution and care!

Special Challenges in Transferring

You may need to move residents who present special challenges and require two or more people in transferring. They may be residents who...

1. cannot bear weight on at least one strong leg. This may be a resident who has contractures of both legs, has both legs amputated, is paralyzed from the neck down (quadriplegic) or paralyzed from the waist down (paraplegic) or is unconscious.

2. are fearful, anxious or combative.

3. have tubes attached, are in casts, or are in traction.

4. are overweight

Assistive devices are helpful in moving residents and can make your job safer and easier. Some assistance devices are:

Gait or Transfer Belt - This is a device to help people who are weak or unsteady on their feet. It is called a transfer belt when you are assisting people in a transfer, such as from bed to chair. It is called a gait belt when it is used to assist in walking.

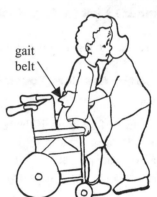

Do not use a gait belt on residents who are pregnant, have had a recent abdominal wound or abdominal surgery, have a gastrostomy tube in the stomach, or a colostomy.

Apply the gait belt over clothing, never against bare skin. Apply the gait belt under breasts.

gait belt

The belt should be snug; not too loose, not too tight. You should be able to put 2-3 fingers between the belt and the resident.

Buckle the belt securely and for comfort position the buckle to the side not over the spine. Follow the manufactures directions for gait belt use.

Hold the belt with an underhand grasp, one hand on each side of the resident.

Mechanical Lift also called **Hoyer Lift**

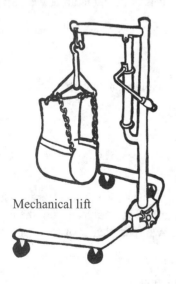

Mechanical lift

A Mechanical lift is a device that can move residents who are very heavy and/ or helpless and cannot be safely moved by caregivers alone. It can be used to move residents in and out of beds, wheelchairs, tubs, whirlpools, etc. It requires two caregivers to perform this procedure safely. You must be trained how to use the specific lift.

Procedure: Use of a Mechanical Lift

1. Lock the wheels on the bed.

2. Raise the bed to a height that is conducive to good body mechanics for the caregiver.

3. Lower the head of the bed to a flat position if the resident can tolerate this.

4. One caregiver stands on each side of the bed.

5. Lower the bedrails.

6. Roll the resident toward one caregiver and position the sling under his/her body. The sling should extend from the resident's upper shoulders to behind the knees (follow the manufacturers instructions). Roll the resident onto his/her back.

7. Position the resident in a Semi-Fowlers position.

8. Lower the bed to its lowest level.

9. Position the lift over the person and lock the lift wheels in position.

10. Lock the wheelchair brakes.

11. Attach the sling to the swivel bar.

12. Raise the lift until the resident and sling is suspended above the bed.

13. Support the resident's legs as the sling is moved away from the bed to the chair.

14. Position the resident in the lift over the wheelchair and gently lower the person into the chair.

15. Unhook the sling.

16. Check the resident for comfort. Cover the persons lap with a lap blanket.

17. Leave the signaling device within reach.

Slide Boards - Helpful in "bridging the gap" in moving the resident from bed to stretcher or gurney. They can also be used for residents who cannot bear weight by standing. A slide board can be put between a bed and a chair. The resident can slide across from one surface to the other.

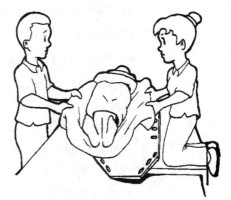

Trapeze Bars - Helpful for residents who have upper extremity strength to move themselves up in bed. This is a metal triangle that is suspended from an overhead frame over the resident. The resident can hold onto this and turn over, or pull self up in bed.

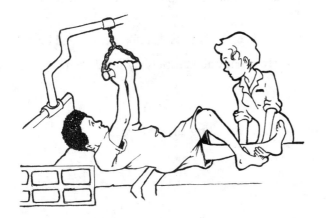

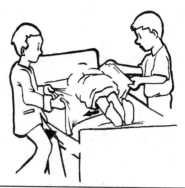

Draw Sheets - This is a half sheet that is placed under the resident from shoulder to thigh. With a care giver on each side of the draw sheet the resident can be lifted up in bed.

Be sure to do the following before any procedures with the resident.
- ◆ Knock on the door before entering the room.
- ◆ Introduce yourself.
- ◆ Explain the procedure, speaking clearly while facing the resident at his/her eye level.
- ◆ Pull the curtain, screen, or close the door for privacy.
- ◆ Wash your hands

Procedure: Turning A Resident In Bed Away From You (One Person)

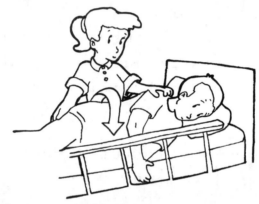

1. Adjust the bed to a proper working height for you (waist or hip level).

2. Make sure the bed is flat.

3. Lower the rail on your side of the bed, raise the rail on the far side.

4. While the resident lies on back, move the shoulder closest to you and then the leg closest to you.

5. Move the resident's farthest arm to head and cross the closest arm across chest.

6. Place one hand on their shoulder and the other on their hip. Turn the resident toward the raised side rail.

7. Place pillows under the upper arm, leg and head of the resident for comfort and support.

8. Check for the resident's comfort and correct body alignment (they should be lying in a straight line).

9. Put up remaining side rail.

10. Return the bed to the lowest position and leave call signal within reach.

11. Wash your hands.

Procedure: Assisting the Resident to Turn Toward You: (One Person) and Positioning Resident on their Side

1. Adjust the bed to a proper height for you (waist or hip level).

2. Make sure the bed is flat.

3. Lower the rail on your side, raise the rail on the far side.

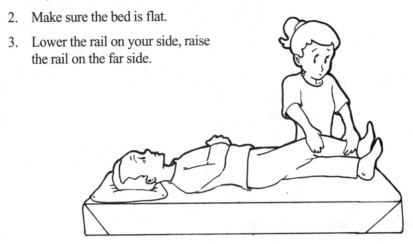

4. While the resident is lying on back, first move the shoulder then the leg closer to you.

5. Raise the rail closest to you. Go to the other side of the bed and lower the rail.

6. Raise the resident's closest arm to his/her head and place the other arm across the chest. Cross the resident's leg farthest from you over the other leg.

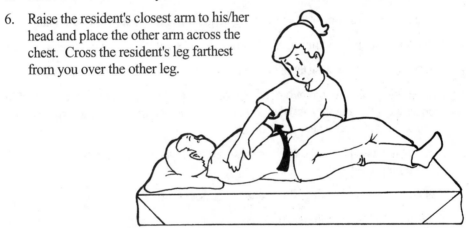

7. Place one hand on the resident's shoulder and the other on his/her hip. Turn the resident toward you on his/her side.

8. Place a pillow under the upper arm for support and one under the upper leg with hip in proper alignment. Insure proper alignment...

    ■ head supported on pillow

    ■ shoulder adjusted so resident is not lying on arm

    ■ back supported by pillow

    ■ top knee flexed, knee and ankle supported

9. Check for comfort. Cover resident with top linen.

10. Lower the bed to its lowest level and leave the call signal within easy reach.

11. Wash your hands.

Moving a Resident to the Side of the Bed

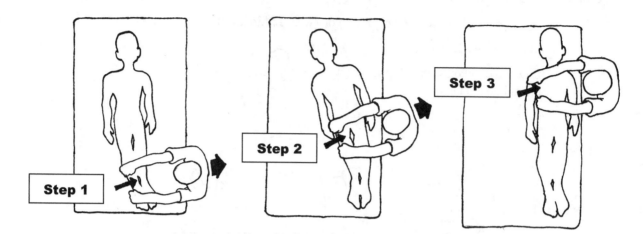

Procedure: Log-Rolling A Resident In Bed

Log rolling means turning a resident, keeping the head, back and legs in a straight line. This may be necessary if the resident may have neck and back problems or has had back or hip surgery.

1. Lock bed wheels.

2. Raise the bed to a comfortable working height and make sure the bed is flat.

3. Place the resident on a turning sheet, on their back with a pillow between their legs.

4. Position two nursing assistants on the left side of the bed and one on the right.

5. On the count of three, the two nursing assistants on the left side roll the resident toward themselves. The nursing assistant on the right rolls the resident away from self. The turning sheet is used as an aid in rolling.

6. The nursing assistant at the head makes sure the head and neck remain in a straight line and are supported.

7. Position the resident with pillows and check for comfort.

8. Place the call light within reach.

9. Wash you hands.

Procedure: Repositioning a Resident in a Wheelchair:

1. Lock the wheelchair brakes.

2. Raise the footrests or turn them out of the way.

3. Stand behind the resident.

4. While keeping your back straight and bending with your knees, place your arms around the resident's torso, under their arms.

5. Lift the resident placing their hips against the back of the chair.

6. Make sure the resident is comfortable.

7. Put footrests in proper position with resident's feet resting on footrests.

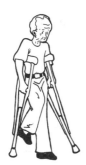

♦ **Crutches** - This should only be used as prescribed for the resident and fitted correctly according to the resident's height. The crutches need to be in good repair, with the rubber tips in good condition. The resident also needs to be trained in how to use the crutches properly by the physical or occupational therapist. The weight should be on the hand bars and not on underarms as the resident ambulates.

♦ **Walker** - This is a lightweight metal frame with four rubber tipped legs or two legs and two wheels. The walker should be an appropriate height for the resident and a physical therapist should teach the resident how to use it properly. The resident needs to raise the walker upward, set it down fully with all four legs touching the ground completely and then walk. The walker should be moved 10-18 inches at a time.

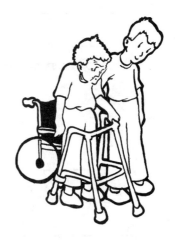

Chapter 7 - Quiz Yourself

True or False

1. _____ If a resident has a right sided weakness or paralysis, put the chair you will be transferring to, on the right side.

2. _____ A resident can bear weight on their contractured leg.

3. _____ A resident's position should be changed every 4 hours.

4. _____ It is safe to put all residents in a prone position.

5. _____ If residents cannot bear weight on at least one leg, they require a two person transfer.

6. _____ When lifting, you should stand with your feet together, bending at the waist while keeping your knees locked.

7. _____ It is acceptable for the residents to put their arms around your neck as you transfer them.

8. _____ A Fowler's position is sitting up in bed at a 45° angle.

9. Name 5 assistive devices that can help you move the difficult to move resident.

_____   _____

_____   _____

_____

10. What are the 3 natural curves in the back that should be maintained at all times?

_____   _____

_____

11. Define what the term "poor body mechanics" means.

_____

_____

12. Name 5 important rules of good body mechanics.

_____

_____

_____

_____

_____

13. Name different types of residents with special needs who may present challenges in lifting.

_____

_____

14. Name at least 3 instances when it is necessary to have two people assist with lifting.

_____

_____

_____

Chapter 8
Infection Control

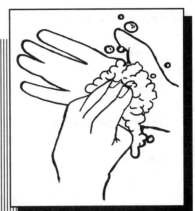

Learning Objectives

1. Explain what microorganisms are and how they are spread

2. Describe an environment that is conducive to bacteria growth

3. List at least 4 instances when hands must be washed on the job

4. Demonstrate proper hand hygiene technique

5. Explain the infectious process and how the cycle can be interrupted

6. Describe the principle of standard precautions

7. List 2 examples each of bacteria and virus

8. Demonstrate proper donning and removing of gown, gloves, and mask

9. Describe how linen should be handled to avoid infection

10. List at least 4 body fluids

11. Explain under what conditions a health care worker should "call in sick"

12. Explain how tuberculosis is transmitted

13. Explain what MRSA is

14. Describe what health care associated infections are and what can be done to prevent them

15. Describe the following: contact, droplet, and airborne precautions

Terms to Know

airborne precautions
asepsis
asymptomatic
bacteria
blood borne pathogen
body fluids
clean
communicable disease
contact precautions
dirty
disinfect
droplet precautions
health care associated infections
immunity
infection
isolation
medical asepsis techniques
microorganisms
MRSA
pathogen
personal protective equipment
standard precautions
sterilize
tuberculosis
vaccination
virus

Terms to Know

Asepsis	to be free of microorganisms (germs)
Aseptic	without infection, germ free
Asymptomatic	absence of symptoms
Bacteria	microorganisms such as E. Coli, streptococcus, staphylococcus, etc.
Blood borne pathogen	disease causing microorganism transmitted by blood, such as Hepatitis B and human immunodeficiency virus (HIV)
Body fluids	blood, semen, vaginal secretions, sputum, saliva, wound drainage, etc.
Clean	uncontaminated
Communicable disease	disease that can be transmitted (passed on) from one person to another.
Contaminated	soiled, unclean
Dirty	contaminated, soiled
Disinfect	the process of destroying disease causing organisms.
HBV	Hepatitis B, a blood borne pathogen that causes liver damage.
HIV	Human immunodeficiency virus - the virus that causes AIDS.
Infection	a condition in which the body or part of it is invaded with a pathogen and which causes illness. Signs and symptoms are redness, fever, drainage, soreness, and so on.
Immunity	protection against a certain disease.
Isolation	to separate a person with communicable illness from a well person.
Medical asepsis	techniques to decrease spread of microorganisms.

Microorganism	a living thing that can be seen by a microscope only.
Pathogen	disease causing microorganism
Personal protective equipment	gloves, gowns, masks, goggles, face shields
Sterilize	to destroy all microorganisms. Sterile technique is used during surgery and during some medical procedures.
Standard precautions	a system of infectious disease control which assumes that every direct contact with body fluids is infectious.
Superbugs	antibiotic resistant bacteria
Vaccination	giving a preparation containing weak or dead microorganisms to produce protection against a disease.
Vancomycin Resistant Enterococci (VRE)	a bacteria. It has become resistant to the antibiotic Vancomycin.
Virus	microorganism that lives on a living cell. Examples: common cold, HBV, HIV. It is smaller than bacteria.

Abbreviations to Know

HBV	Hepatitis B Virus
HIV	Human immunodeficiency virus
MRSA	Methycillin resistant staphylococcus aureus
TB	Tuberculosis
URI	upper respiratory infection
UTI	urinary tract infection
VRE	Vancomycin Resistant Enterococci

Infection Control - The Responsibility is Ours!

In the health care setting we need to be aware of **communicable diseases,** diseases that can be transmitted from person to person. Caution and understanding of microorganisms and their spread can help in keeping ourselves healthy. Additionally, proper aseptic techniques can help decrease the risk of spreading communicable diseases from one to another. We all need to be responsible for our own well being as well as that of our residents.

What Causes Disease?

There is a whole invisible world of organisms that can only be seen by a microscope. They are called **microorganisms**. Some are helpful to us, others cause disease. Disease causing microorganisms are called **pathogens**.

Health care associated infections, also known as nosocomial infections, are infections that occur once a patient is in a hospital or a nursing home. Patients are already in a physically vulnerable state due to chronic illness or debilitated condition, therefore are very susceptible to pathogens.

Every year 120,000 patients die of these infections. The most common health care associated infections are urinary tract infections, surgical wound infections, pneumonias, bloodstream infections and MRSA.

The most common way for infection to occur is for bacteria or viruses to enter the persons body during treatment. These organisms can enter through body openings such as through I.V.'s, breathing tubes, surgical wounds, or urinary catheters. Infection is more likely to occur in the person who has a compromised immune system. People who have a compromised immune system frequently are older people, AIDS patients, those on chemotherapy and people who have had invasive procedures like surgery, catheterization, I.V.'s, and people in generally poor health.

Health care workers can easily transmit communicable disease from person to person by not using **aseptic techniques** like hand washing, using gloves, and not using sterile techniques during invasive procedures, etc.. The health care worker who does not consistently wash hands between patients is one of the major causes of infections. All health care workers have a very serious responsibility to carefully and consistently practice good aseptic techniques. Your patients welfare and life depends on it!

Microorganisms can be spread through blood, feces, respiratory droplets (such as by coughing and sneezing) or coming in contact with nasal drainage or wound. Different microorganisms are transmitted by different means. The following are some examples.

Through feces...   hepatitis A, poliomyelitis, E. Coli

Through respiratory droplets...   diphtheria, chicken pox, influenza, meningitis, mononucleosis, pertussis (whopping cough), pneumonia, tuberculosis

Through blood...   HIV, HBV

Different types of microorganisms

BACTERIA - grows best in an environment that is warm ($50\text{-}110^0 F$), moist, and dark. The human body is great for bacteria growth. Bacteria is the most common cause of infection in the health care environment. Some bacteria require oxygen for their survival, other bacteria do not. Some common illnesses caused by bacteria are: bladder infections caused by e coli, strep throat caused by streptococcus, tuberculosis, some types of pneumonia, and skin infections caused by staphylococcus aureus.

Staphylococcus aureus is frequently present on the skin but when it enters the body, through a cut for example, it may cause a localized infection with symptoms of redness, localized heat, soreness, fluid-filled blisters, large painful bumps under the skin and purulent (pus) drainage. If not promptly treated with antibiotics, the infection can go throughout the entire body and be deadly.

Methicillin Resistant Staphylococcus Aureus (MRSA) is a serious infection that can become life threatening if not treated. There are indeed thousands of people who die of MRSA annually. The Center for Disease Control now states that more people die of MRSA than AIDS in the U.S..Previously MRSA was found mostly in hospitals and nursing homes. It now is found in prisons, schools, and in the general community. Any one can get MRSA and infect other people.

MRSA is a staph bacteria that lives on the skin or in the nose. It has become resistant to many antibiotics over the years because people have used antibiotics inappropriately, that is stopping antibiotics early, missing doses or taking them without a prescription. This has resulted in a stronger bacteria, or a "super bug" that is harder to treat.

MRSA can appear as any of the following skin infections: fluid filled blisters, large red painful bumps or boils, swollen hot pus filled cut, or a reddened area that looks like an insect bite.

More seriously, MRSA can be in other parts of the body such as the eyes, lungs, urine and blood. If you have any of the above skin infections, contact your physician immediately.

You can get MRSA by touching someone with MRSA or something that has MRSA on it, such as towels, clothes, athletic equipment, door knobs, phones, etc.. It can survive on surfaces for months. If you touch a contaminated surface and bring it to your eyes, nose, or pick it up through a cut in your skin, you can become infected. Good hygiene with frequent hand washing, keeping any open skin areas covered, and generally maintaining a healthy immune system is beneficial.

Vancomycin Resistant Enterococcus (VRE) is a bacteria that has become resistant to the antibiotic Vancomycin and many other antibiotics. It is the leading cause of surgical wound infections, UTI and bacteremia. Transmission can occur by coming into contact with blood, stool and urine infected with VRE. Healthcare workers can transmit it on their hands. Direct contact with equipment or contaminated environmental surfaces is another way for VRE transmission.

Clostridium Difficile, also known as C. Dif is a spore-forming bacteria that is found in people who are healthy or ill. When a person is healthy, millions of good bacteria keep C. Dif in check. When a person takes antibiotics, good bacteria level is decreased and C. Dif can over populate in the intestines. Toxins are created which cause ulcerations resulting in diarrhea, cramping and later weakness, dehydration, vomiting and blood in feces. G.I. tract surgery may increase the risk of developing the disease also. C. Dif is mostly only contagious from person to person through the fecal-oral route. It is spread by spores in feces. Avoid direct contact with the infected person's feces and anything it may have touched such as linen, bedpans, toilets, clothing, etc..

VIRUS - very small organisms that can survive only in other living cells. There are many viruses with the following only being a few.

HIV - human immunodeficiency virus   HBV - hepatitis B virus

Measles   Influenza

Microorganisms can be everywhere! They can be in food, on animals, on objects, in waste, in the air, or in liquids.

The body has two lines of defense against infection. These are...

External defense - skin prevents microorganisms from entering the body. Any breaks in the skin can be entry points for microorganisms.

Internal defense - white blood cells in the blood to fight off disease causing microorganisms once they have entered the body.

For an infection to be passed on the following factors must be present.

Infectious Agent - the pathogen. Examples: staph, strep, etc..

Reservoir - the place where growth and reproduction takes place. Example: A person with a disease.

Portal of exit - how the pathogen leaves the reservoir. Examples: Open area on skin (no matter how small), draining wounds, urine, feces, blood, respiratory droplets, etc.

Means of Transmission - how the pathogen goes from the portal of exit to the entry site. Example: On hands, on food, sewage, etc..

Portal of Entry - the way the pathogen gets into the new host or receiver of the organism. Examples: Through skin, nose, cuts, mouth, urinary catheter, blood, food, mucous membranes, etc.

Susceptible Host - someone more likely to become infected, such as a person who has poor nutrition, has chronic debilitating illness, has poor hygiene, has respiratory and/or circulatory disease, lives in crowded situations.

The examples listed above are only some examples. Many more exist.

The following are possible signs of infection...

lack of appetite	rapid pulse	elevated temperature	redness, swelling
diarrhea	unusual discharge	nausea or vomiting	fatigue
difficulty breathing	lack of appetite	chills	pain
confusion	muscle aches	heat or warmth of a body part	
foul smelling, cloudy urine			

Interrupting the Cycle

Things you can do to break the cycle of infection...

Proper hand hygiene and use of gloves

Practice good hygiene for yourself and your resident

Handle linen properly

Good housekeeping; separating clean from dirty.

Take good care of yourself with good nutrition and rest

Do not report to work if you are ill.

Cover any open areas on your skin

Immunizations including HBV vaccine

Consistent use of standard precautions

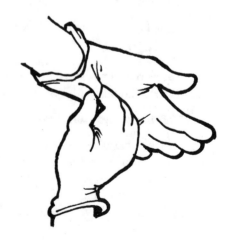

You should not go to work if...

> You are coughing, sneezing and have a sore throat.

> Your body aches with sore muscles.

> You have elevated temperature.

If you have questions about your health and reporting to work, check with your charge nurse. Avoid infecting vulnerable residents!

Standard Precautions

Many diseases have **asymptomatic** periods of time when a person exhibits no signs or symptoms of illness but can communicate the disease. For example, a person with Hepatitis B may look well and feel well for 6 months prior to becoming ill. During those asymptomatic months they however could pass on the virus to others through non-protected sex, or exposure to blood. For a person who is HIV positive this asymptomatic stage is 10 years during which they can infect others through specific means. We therefore cannot rely on outward signs and symptoms as an indication of illness.

In 1996 the Center for Disease Control implemented a new set of guidelines to decrease spread of disease. The purpose is to protect health care workers from the resident's microorganisms and to prevent the spread of microorganisms and infection to others. Standard precautions were developed to replace the previously used universal precautions. **Universal precautions** pertained to body fluids that contained visible blood. Standard precautions now pertain to ALL body fluids, with or without visible blood.

The principle of standard precautions is to assume that all patients are infectious. By adhering to precautions, health care workers are protected in all interactions. The Center for Disease Control defines **standard precautions** as:

"a system of infectious disease control which assumes that every direct contact with body fluids is infectious, and requires every employee exposed to direct contact with body fluids to be protected as though such body fluids were infected with a blood-borne pathogen. (HIV/HBV are only two of many blood-borne pathogens)."

Standard precautions must be practiced when you may come in contact with...

- ◆ blood
- ◆ all body fluids (except sweat)
- ◆ non-intact skin
- ◆ mucus membranes (moist lining of mouth, nose, eyes, genital area)

Respiratory hygiene / cough etiquette

Cover your mouth and nose when coughing or sneezing to contain respiratory secretions. Do not cough or sneeze into your hands. To avoid spreading microorganisms, cough into the inside of your elbow or use a tissue. Dispose the tissue into a waste container and wash your hands.

Transmission Based Precautions (used in addition to standard precautions)

Residents who are known or suspected to be infectious may in addition to standard precautions require one or more of the following...

Contact Precautions - for residents who may transmit a microorganism by touch of an infected area such as open wounds or drainage. Examples are skin diseases resulting in skin breaks, and conjunctivitis (pink eye), etc. Avoid touching any body drainage directly or objects that may have come in contact with the drainage such as clothing and linen. Wear gown and gloves while touching the resident directly such as transferring, bathing and while handling potentially contaminated linen.

Droplet Precautions - for residents infected by microorganisms transmitted by droplets that travel through the air within 3 feet of the resident when they cough, laugh, sneeze or talk. Examples are diphtheria and influenza. A private room is desirable but if not available, place with another resident with a similar microorganism. Door to the room may remain open. Gloves and gowns should be worn with all contact. Wear mask and eyewear when working within 3 feet of the resident.

Airborne Precautions - for residents who are infected with microorganisms transmitted by airborne nuclei such as tuberculosis, chicken pox, and measles. These organisms are tiny and can travel long distances on dust particles and moisture in the air. Residents require private rooms with the door closed at all times. Special rooms with special air handling and ventilation are required. The staff must wear special respirators when entering the room. Gown and gloves should be used for all contact.

Personal protective equipment (PPE)

Gloves

Gloves should be worn when there is potential for direct skin contact with...

- Blood

- Infectious materials such as wound drainage.

- Contaminated items like soiled linen or clothing, tissues, undergarments, etc.

- Body fluids like urine, saliva, etc.

- Mucous membranes

Wear gloves when doing the following procedures...

- Perineal care

- Collecting specimens

- Oral care

- Shaving a resident

- Changing colostomy or ileostomy bags

Hold your hands lower than your elbows while scrubbing so water runs down the arms and hands.

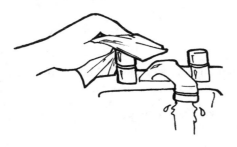

Rinse well

Dry your wrists and hands with a paper towel starting at your fingertips.

Use the paper towel to turn off the faucet to avoid contaminating your clean hands.

Discard the paper towel into a wastebasket.

Frequent hand washing with soap can dry your hands which can cause breaks in the skin. Breaks in the skin are ideal areas for pathogens to enter. Use lotions to moisturize your skin to avoid dryness. Waterless alcohol based hand cleaners are less irritating to the skin than frequent washing with soap. Alcohol based hand rubs are also approved for hand decontamination by the Center for Disease Control. They are used without water so can be quickly used anywhere. If your hands are visibly soiled with blood, other body fluids or dirt, you must use soap and water to thoroughly wash your hands.

Points to Remember

You are protecting not only yourself from coming in direct contact with body fluids but also other residents who you will come in contact with, to whom you can pass on the contamination. You therefore must do the following **between** each resident...

> discard any gloves, gown or mask
>
> wash your hands

Each resident should have their own supplies and equipment which should not be shared with others. This includes bedpans, urinals, commodes, wash basins, emesis basins, soap, toothbrushes, combs, etc.. Do not take equipment from one room to another.

Tuberculosis

We are increasingly aware of tuberculosis (TB) because recently there has been a resurgence of its occurrence. Worldwide, 3 million people die of TB annually. In the 1950's TB was greatly decreased due to development of powerful antibiotics. Since the mid 1980's however, there has been a dramatic increase in the incidence of TB. If you are exposed to someone who has active TB you do not necessarily get active TB. You may acquire dormant, latent TB infection. For those infected with dormant, latent TB, there is a 10% chance they will develop active TB in their lifetime. One third of the world's population is infected with latent TB. Active TB is a serious but treatable disease. Know your TB status, get tested.

What is it?

Tuberculosis is caused by the airborne mycobacterium tuberculosis, a bacteria that can be spread from person to person through the air. Tiny, invisible droplets travel through the air when an infected person laughs, coughs, sneezes or possibly just speaks. It can infect anyone in close proximity especially if they are repeatedly exposed or are in small, confined spaces with a person with active TB. Only a small fraction of those infected develop active TB as long as the person has a well functioning immune system. If, however, the immune system is not doing its job, the germ will multiply with the body producing enzymes that are toxic to the lungs and other organs. Most but not all TB strains can be treated with drugs.

Who Is At Risk?

◆ People with a suppressed immune system, such as people with AIDS or people who use medications that suppress the immune system such as corticosteroids.

◆ Homeless people who may have poor nutrition and unhygienic living environments.

◆ People from countries with high TB rates.

◆ Healthcare professionals who work around TB.

◆ The elderly.

◆ People with chronic, debilitating illness.

◆ Alcoholics and intravenous drug users.

Know Your TB Status!

The TB skin test can tell you if the tuberculosis bacteria is in your body. A small amount of solution is injected under the skin by a health care professional. The injection site needs to be examined by a health care professional in 48-72 hours who observes for a skin reaction. A reddened, raised area means a "positive" reaction. This does not necessarily mean a person has active TB, but means a person has the TB infection in their body. A "positive" reaction should be followed up by a chest x-ray for a definitive diagnosis.

Active TB Disease

A chest x-ray would identify active TB. TB disease means the TB bacteria is present in the body, multiplying and likely spreading to other people. Symptoms include a chronic cough, coughing up blood, poor appetite, weight loss, and fever. If untreated, tuberculosis can be deadly. It can affect the lungs, brain, and kidneys.

How is Active TB Treated?

Taking medications as prescribed is vital! Treatment will take months and directions must be carefully followed. Medications should not be discontinued even if there are no symptoms until the physician approves termination of medications.

Chapter 8 - Quiz Yourself

True or False

1. _____ The human body is an excellent environment for bacteria growth.

2. _____ Tuberculosis is spread through the air.

3. _____ Asymptomatic period of time means a period of time when the person shows no signs or symptoms of disease.

4. _____ After washing your hands, turn the faucet off with your bare hands.

5. _____ It is not necessary to wash your hands after removing your gloves.

6. _____ Many people die unnecessarily of health care associated infections. We must all do our part in decreasing those infections.

7. _____ When carrying linen, clutch it close to your body.

8. _____ It is alright to put dirty laundry on the resident's overbed table.

9. _____ It is acceptable to throw dirty laundry on the floor.

10. _____ A person is more likely to pass microorganisms from one person to another on their hands.

Fill in the correct answers.

11. Name 3 instances when hands must be washed on the job.

_____

_____

_____

12. List 3 medical aseptic techniques you can use on the job.

_____

_____

_____

Circle the one correct answer

13. The body fluid that is of greatest risk for transmitting deadly pathogens is...

    a.   sputum
    b.   saliva
    c.   blood
    d.   perspiration

14. Standard precautions should be used...

    a.   only when the patient exhibits signs and symptoms of illness.
    b.   in all interactions when direct contact with body fluids is possible.
    c.   only when a diagnosis of communicable disease is made.

15. Mucus membranes are...

    a.   body fluids.
    b.   moist lining of mouth, nose, eyes, genital areas.
    c.   over bony areas.

16. You should not go to work if...

    a.   you are tired.
    b.   your are coughing, sneezing and have elevated temperature.
    c.   you have flu symptoms.
    d.   b and c

Chapter 9

Blood Borne Pathogens
HIV and HBV

Learning Objectives

1. Give 2 examples of blood borne pathogens.

2. Describe the immune system and how it helps keep us healthy.

3. Explain the difference between HIV and AIDS.

4. Describe the 3 stages of HIV/AIDS and what the symptoms are for each.

5. Explain how HIV is transmitted.

6. List at least 3 risk factors for HIV.

7. Name 3 things you can do to avoid becoming infected with HIV.

8. Describe what an opportunistic disease is and name at least 3 of them.

9. Explain some psychological issues a person with HIV/AIDS would have while coping with this illness.

10. Explain what Hepatitis B is, how it is transmitted and why it is of great concern especially to health care givers.

11. Describe what health care givers can do to minimize risk of becoming infected with blood borne pathogens.

Terms to Know

hepatitis A, B, C
HIV
HBV
asymptomatic
blood borne pathogen
opportunistic disease
immune system
AIDS

What Happens When Someone Becomes Infected?

Within 1-2 weeks after exposure to the HIV infection, the infected person may develop flu-like symptoms that last a few days and go away. The person is infectious to others from the time they themselves are infected. Not everyone exposed to HIV becomes infected.

Meanwhile Inside the Body. . .

Immediately upon infection, thousands of HIV particles are reproducing themselves in the white blood cells called helper T cells. They are known as CD4 cells, the linchpin of the immune system.

Stages of HIV Infection

1. **Asymptomatic stage** (no signs, no symptoms) may last an average of ten years. The person may look and feel well and have no idea they are ill. Women seem to have generally a shorter asymptomatic stage for as yet unknown reasons. The person continues to be able to infect others. Some people have remained asymptomatic for more than fifteen years and researchers are studying them to see what can be learned about keeping others healthy longer.

   Meanwhile Inside the Body...

   The virus is now swept from the blood and is in the lymph nodes. The virus continues to replicate itself (copies and duplicates itself). In the meantime the body fights powerfully: antibodies move through the blood neutralizing HIV particles, and specialized white blood cells called killer T cells attack and destroy infected tissue. Soon more HIV particles escape from the lymph nodes into the blood and the immune system becomes weaker and helper T cells start to die. The HIV test can detect the presence of HIV antibodies (our bodies response to the presence of HIV) usually within 6 months of being infected.

2. **Symptomatic stage** may last many months. The symptoms may be nightsweats, nausea, extreme fatigue, diarrhea, severe weight loss, etc. The person is feeling very, very ill but may improve temporarily and then symptoms return or change. It is difficult to maintain a normal work and activity level during this stage.

   Meanwhile Inside the Body...

   The helper T cell count drops from 1,000 cells per milliliter of blood to less than 500. The immune system continues to deteriorate.

3. The **diagnosis of AIDS** is made officially when the helper T cells count falls below 200. It is in this stage that the person falls victim to a variety of opportunistic diseases. The course is unpredictable, the person may battle different opportunistic diseases, recover temporarily and fall victim to another. The Center for Disease Control states that average life expectancy is 22 years and most people with medication and treatment may live out their normal life span.

   Meanwhile Inside the Body...

   The amount of helper T cells plummet so the body cannot muster a fight against the HIV invasion. The person dies of an opportunistic disease. See the list of opportunistic diseases later in this chapter.

You can become infected with HIV in the following ways...

♦ Having sexual intercourse - anal, vaginal or oral with an infected person.

♦ Sharing drug needles or syringes (drug users)

♦ Coming in direct contact with infected blood such as being splashed in the face, eyes or mouth with infected blood, or touching infected blood directly.

Also. . .

♦ Women infected with HIV can pass it on to their babies during pregnancy, during birth or while breast feeding. If women are treated during pregnancy, less than 3% of the babies will become infected.

♦ People who received infected blood transfusions, particularly hemophiliacs prior to 1985. After 1985, blood has been carefully screened and the risk now is quite low.

How It Is NOT Transmitted

The AIDS virus is transmitted only by close, intimate contact in a very specific manner. You cannot get it by casual contact! For example, the following are ways you **cannot** get HIV...

♦ Sitting next to someone who is infected

♦ Sharing telephones, office supplies and equipment

♦ Sitting next to an infected person on the bus or in a theatre

♦ Touching door knobs

♦ Using same bathroom facilities as an infected person

♦ Being served by someone who has HIV/AIDS or eating food prepared by someone who has HIV/AIDS

♦ Being bitten by mosquitoes

♦ Touching or hugging an infected person

♦ Sharing forks, spoons, knives or drinking glasses

Where does the virus live?

The virus lives in body fluids transmitted through blood, semen and vaginal fluids.

How does the AIDS virus enter the body?

♦ When syringes or needles are shared by drug users, the virus can enter the bloodstream through a puncture made by a needle containing contaminated blood. This is a very effective way to transmit the virus.

♦ During sexual activity, the virus contained in the blood, semen or vaginal fluid of an infected person enters the body of another through the penis, vagina, mouth or rectum.

Unprotected Sex is Dangerous

HIV can be in semen (including the first drop of fluid even before ejaculation) and in vaginal fluids. HIV can enter the body through the vagina, penis, rectum and when engaging in oral sex, through the mouth. Anal sex is risky for both males and females.

Safe sex is no sex. The next best thing is "safer" sex which means use of a latex condom. Several important facts to remember about condom use are:

- Use condoms consistently, each time there is sexual activity and before the first drops of semen.

- Use only latex condoms. Natural animal skin condoms are more porous and may allow the virus to pass.

- Use only water-based lubricants. Never use oil based lubricants like Vaseline, mineral or cooking oil or cold cream.

Could You Be At Risk?

The AIDS virus is transmitted frequently through unsafe sex practices. When you have sex with someone you also in a sense are having sex with every one of that person's past partners. Your partner may have gotten infected in the past and he or she could unknowingly pass the virus to you. How well do you know your partner? Here are some questions you should ask yourself:

- Am I sure my sexual partner does not presently have HIV?

- How sure is my sexual partner about his or her sexual partners, dating back to 1970 or beginning of their sexual activity?

- Has my sexual partner used IV drugs (street use) or received blood transfusions or blood products since the 1970's?

- Did my sexual partner have a previous sex partner who used IV drugs?

- Did my sexual partner ever engage in high risk behaviors such as anal intercourse or had sex with male or female prostitutes?

Additionally you may want to ask yourself if you or your sexual partners have engaged in any of the following since 1978?

- Had oral, anal or vaginal intercourse without a condom with anyone else besides a regular sex partner?

- Had multiple sex partners?

- Had (STD's) sexually transmitted diseases? STD's include herpes, syphilis, gonorrhea, chlamydia, etc. The same type of high risk activity that infected a person with a STD may also put them at risk of becoming infected with HIV. Additionally some STD's cause open genital areas which can more easily become infected with HIV.

- Been exposed to the blood or body fluids of a person infected with the AIDS virus?

If you answer "yes," "maybe" or "don't know" to any of these questions you may have been exposed and become infected. You may want to get tested to determine your HIV status. This is especially important if you are starting a sexual relationship or are considering pregnancy.

If you find your results are negative (you do not have HIV) you can relax and rest easy. Of course continue "safer" sex techniques in your everyday life.

If a person finds they are positive (they have the HIV infection) it is important to be under a physicians care and take good care of oneself. Additionally, as always practice techniques to prevent transmission of HIV to others.

Before starting a sexual relationship, it would be wise for both partners to be tested for AIDS antibodies. Remember that it would take up to six months for the antibodies to show up in the blood after a person was infected. A long-term, monogamous (faithful) relationship with an uninfected partner would put you at low or no risk for HIV infections.

HIV and Drug Use

Injecting drugs can spread HIV from one person to another when injection equipment is shared or re-used by another person. HIV may be found in a variety of items used for drug injection, including needles, syringes, cotton, etc.

If you use drugs, seek help to help you stop! Drug abuse programs can be very helpful. If you cannot stop immediately do not share any needles "works" equipment. All sterile disposable supplies should be used once only. Call 1-800-342-AIDS for more information on Drugs and HIV.

All syringes, needles, I.V.'s etc. used in clinics, doctors offices and hospitals by professional medical personnel of course are safe. Sterile, disposable equipment is used once only and is safe.

Giving blood for transfusions is of course also totally safe.

What are precautions you can take?

♦ Education

♦ Know the truth and consistently practice precautions

♦ Know your sexual partner.

♦ Remember the person could be infectious but look well and feel well. Don't expect any outward signs!

♦ Know your partner's sexual history. Having sex with someone is like having sex with their previous partners, and their partner's partners, etc.. It is hard to be absolutely sure of your partners sexual history.

♦ Know your partner's current and previous history of I.V. drug use. (25% of I.V. drug users are HIV positive)

♦ Avoid anal intercourse. There is a high risk of infection because delicate rectal lining is likely to have small rips and tears with anal intercourse. This creates access into the blood stream. If one of the partners is infected, HIV can pass between semen and blood.

♦ Get tested!

♦ Practice "safer sexual practices" such as consistently and properly using latex condoms. Proper use of condoms gives a high degree of protection but no sex is the only guarantee of no risk.

♦ Being in a mutually monogamous sexual relationship with a person who is not HIV positive.

♦ Do not share intravenous syringes and needles.

♦ Avoid use of alcohol. Alcohol generally lowers immunity and increases risk of becoming infected. Alcohol lowers inhibitions and affects judgment. A person under the influence of alcohol may make poor choices regarding sexual behavior.

♦ Women should know their HIV status before becoming pregnant. HIV can be passed to the fetus, but this risk can be dramatically reduced if the pregnant mother is treated.

Follow up to Exposure to HIV/AIDS

If you experience a "substantial exposure" to another person's blood or potentially infectious material, contact your supervisor immediately. The person to whose blood you have been exposed to, with their consent, should be tested to determine HIV/AIDS status. The health care worker should have HBV/HIV antibody testing immediately and re-tested at 6 weeks, 3 months, and 6 months past exposure. See a physician promptly.

If your eyes are splattered with blood or body fluids, flush your eyes immediately with clean, running water for 5 minutes.

If you are splashed in the mouth with blood or body fluids, rinse your mouth with a 50/50 mix of hydrogen peroxide and water.

If you sustain a needle stick injury, bite, or puncture wound, squeeze the area to cause bleeding. Wash thoroughly with soap and water or pour hydrogen peroxide on the wound.

Outlook for the Future

There is much research going on currently into HIV/ AIDS. There is research into developing vaccines sometime in the future but it is not predicted in the near future. We have improved medications and developed others that have extended the life of people in the AIDS phase. AZT has helped many for a period of time. Unfortunately the virus is notoriously changeable and usually it manages to mutate into a form that is no longer susceptible to AZT or any of the chemical versions ddi, ddc and 3TC. A class of antiviral drugs used now include protease inhibitors which seem to have extended life and caused a drop in level of HIV in the blood. Drugs are used in combination and require careful monitoring during their use. The challenges continue because the virus can and does change. There is no cure. Medications are very expensive. The outlook is cautiously optimistic for the future.

Legal Ethical Issues

HIV infection and AIDS are all considered "handicapping" status in Section 504 of the Federal Rehabilitation Act of 1973. This means it is illegal to discriminate against someone who has AIDS or is HIV infected. It is also illegal to discriminate against someone who is believed to have AIDS or who is believed to be HIV infected, even though that person is not infected, in...

employment

rental, purchase or sale of apartment, house or real estate

places of accommodation (restaurants, theatres, etc.)

health care, legal services and other personal services available to the general public

applying for loan or credit

Persons with HIV and/ or AIDS who feel discriminated against on the basis of handicap may file a complaint with the Office of Civil Rights of the US Dept. of Health and Human Services or Washington State Human Rights Commission.

All medical information about a person who is diagnosed as having HIV or AIDS shall be held in strict confidence. A breach of this confidentiality is illegal. If such a breach occurs, legal action can be taken against the person breaching the confidentiality. A person could be convicted and fined.

Standard Precautions

The Center for Disease Control has made it a requirement that all health care givers use Standard Precautions in all their interactions with residents. If a caregiver consistently uses standard precautions they should be protected from being infected with blood borne pathogens such as hepatitis B and HIV. If you are taking care of someone with HBV, HIV or AIDS there is no higher level of infection control you would need to take. Standard precautions used consistently, that is with every interaction with the resident is your highest level of protection. Carefully review the information listed on standard precautions and infection control earlier in the book.

A very small number of health care workers have been infected on the job usually being stuck with a needle already used on a HIV infected patient. Only 3 out of every 1000 health care workers that have been stuck by needles used on HIV infected patients, themselves become infected. This risk can be reduced if health care workers treat all blood and other body fluids as if it contained HIV.

HIV and Psychological Issues

People living with HIV-AIDS are confronted with many issues that are difficult to handle such as...

- ◆ loss of physical strength
- ◆ possible loss of mental activity
- ◆ loss of a job due to poor health
- ◆ loss of self sufficiency
- ◆ physical weakness and pain
- ◆ anxiety
- ◆ depression in facing a progressive and terminal illness
- ◆ possibly being rejected or discriminated by others due to ignorance and fear
- ◆ sadness and helplessness
- ◆ possible isolation
- ◆ fear of the unknown as the disease progresses
- ◆ high cost of treatment

- possible loss of insurance related to job loss

- physical disfigurement as disease takes its toll

Diseases and Infections Associated with HIV Infection

Some of the "opportunistic" diseases and infections associated with HIV infection are...

- Pneumocystis Carinii Pneumonia (PCP) is a lung infection with common symptoms of dry cough and shortness of breath. This affects 92% of all AIDS patients.

- Kaposi's Sarcoma (KS) is a cancer with common symptoms of pink, purple or brown "spots" or lesions on the skin. This affects about 15% of all AIDS patients.

- Toxoplasmosis is a brain infection with common symptoms of fever, headaches, weakness, confusion, seizures and memory loss.

- Cryptococcol Meningitis attacks the central nervous system with common symptoms of headaches, confusion, nausea, seizures and memory loss.

- Candida Albicans is an yeast infection of the mouth, esophagus or lungs with common symptom of severe diarrhea.

- Mycobacterium Avium Intracellulare is an infection of the respiratory tract with common symptoms of weakness and wasting.

- HIV Encephalopathy or AIDS Dementia infects and damages the cells in the brain and spinal cord with common symptoms of confusion, memory loss, motor control problems, mood swings and seizures. This affects about 35% of all AIDS patients.

- Tuberculosis - the lowered immune system makes the patient susceptible to tuberculosis.

- Cervical Cancer - Many female AIDS patients may develop this.

There are many more opportunistic diseases unfortunately, but these are the most common ones. A person may be affected with one opportunistic disease, be ill and recover. Ultimately one of the opportunistic diseases will be fatal.

Community Resources for HIV AIDS

Center for Disease Control National Aids Hotline: 1-800-232-4636

CDC for Alcohol and Drug Information 1-800-729-6686

Viral Hepatitis

Caused by a virus and results in damage to the liver. The severity can vary from mild symptoms to chronic problems or even death. There are several types of viral hepatitis; A, B, C, D, and E. The one that is of greatest risk to the health care worker is Hepatitis B (HBV).

Hepatitis A

How is it transmitted?

It is transmitted from one person to another by the fecal-oral route. Hepatitis A is present in feces of an infected person. If that person does not wash their hands with soap and water after using the toilet and handles uncooked food, the virus can be transmitted to the person consuming the food. Food handlers should be very careful to wash their hands and clean under their finger nails. It is most contagious before there are any symptoms. To minimize risk to yourself, handle anything contaminated with feces carefully. This means wearing gloves when handling bedpans, rectal thermometers, linen and clothes soiled with feces. Be sure to wash your hands and assist the resident to wash their hands.

What are the symptoms?

15-45 days after you get the virus: sudden lack of energy, diarrhea, nausea, fever, stomach pain, jaundice, and dark urine. Mild cases last 1-2 weeks, more severe cases 4-6 weeks.

Hepatitis B (HBV)

Hepatitis B (HBV) is a serious, potentially life-threatening blood borne pathogen. There are an estimated 1.25 million persons with chronic HBV infection in the US. It is important for you to educate yourself as to what it is, what causes it and most importantly, what you can do to avoid becoming infected. HBV is present in blood and body fluids of infected people. It can be spread by…

- ◆ Unprotected sex

- ◆ Contaminated tools used for tattooing and body piercings

- ◆ Recreational I.V. drug use and sharing of needles

- ◆ Accidental needle stick injuries by health care workers

What is it?

Hepatitis B is a virus that causes damage to the liver and other systems, the severity of which can range from mild to severe to fatal. The liver becomes inflamed and cannot pass bile effectively, which is needed to break down fats. It also cannot detoxify blood of toxic substances as well or store vitamins and sugars as needed. This can lead to chronic (on-going) problems for the rest of your life.

Why is HBV even a greater risk than HIV?

Both HBV and HIV are viruses found in the blood. You have a greater risk of becoming infected with HBV however. HBV is more concentrated in blood than HIV. If you had a needle stick injury, you have a 30 times greater chance of becoming infected with HBV as opposed to HIV. The Hepatitis B virus can survive in dried blood on a surface for up to 7 days.

How is it spread?

It is spread through blood and body fluids that contain blood. This means it can be communicated through sexual contact or through sharing of needles, syringes, or needle works by IV drug users. In the work setting, health care workers can get it through needle stick injuries or other puncture wounds, through breaks in the skin, through splashes of body fluids to mucous membranes (eyes, mouth, nose) or touching a contaminated surface and then touching mucous membranes.

What are the symptoms?

- ◆ Many people infected with HBV show no signs or symptoms. They are however infectious and can pass on HBV to others. 25% will later develop cirrhosis of the liver, liver failure or cancer of the liver. This can happen many years later.

- ◆ Some people may have very mild, flu-like symptoms such as fatigue, achy muscles, fever, sore joints and not even realize that they have developed hepatitis B. They are infectious to others. 10% of people with HBV become carriers and can spread the disease their entire life.

- ◆ Some people may have very debilitating and severe symptoms such as muscle and joint aches, headache, abdominal pain, extreme fatigue and weakness, nausea, vomiting, jaundice (yellowing of the skin and whites of eyes) and it can last weeks or even months.

- ◆ Many people recover completely within 6 months.

- ◆ Some die if they develop acute hepatitis.

- ◆ Symptoms may not appear up to 6 months after infection, however the person is infectious from the time they become infected.

Get vaccinated!

A vaccine is a preparation containing weak or dead microorganisms that is given to a person to produce immunity or protection against a disease. A vaccine for Hepatitis B is available. The vaccine is given in a series of vaccinations over a period of 6 months. The Center for Disease Control recommends that anyone who has potential for contact with blood or body fluids get vaccinated. Speak to your employer about the vaccine. If you suspect an on-the-job exposure, speak to your supervisor right away and contact your doctor. This vaccine is routinely given now to infants and children as immunization. It is hoped that if everyone gets vaccinated, that in one to two generations this disease can be eliminated.

What can I do to protect myself?

Avoid coming in contact with body fluids

Use standard precautions

Get vaccinated

Hepatitis C (Also known as HCV)

Hepatitis C was identified in the late 1980's. About 4 million Americans have Hepatitis C and most people do not know it. A diagnostic antibody test is available to determine if a person has it. Hepatitis C can be cured if treatment is started before serious liver scarring occurs. Often there are no symptoms until the disease becomes severe. It is highly recommended that people get tested to see if they have been infected so life saving treatment can be started in time. Hepatitis C and its complications account for the majority of liver transplants in this country. Hepatitis C can be spread in the same way as Hepatitis B. The symptoms may be fatigue, lack of appetite, stomach pain, nausea and vomiting. Many people will have no symptoms over many years until it causes permanent damage, possibly leading to death. The most common means of transmission is contaminated blood transfusions (especially prior to 1980), needle stick exposure, piercings or tattoes done without proper sterile techniques and recreational intravenous drug use. Hepatitis C is the leading cause of cirrhosis of the liver and liver cancer. In the next few years, the death rate is predicted to surpass annual HIV/AIDS deaths.

Hepatitis D

This is a virus transmitted through blood only in the presence of active Hepatitis B. Complications are chronic liver disease. No vaccine is available.

Hepatitis E

This virus is transmitted from feces to mouth. It is particularly deadly in pregnant women. A vaccine is not available.

Chapter 9 - Quiz Yourself

True Or False

1. _____ AIDS is due to a virus that can be transmitted by casual contact or close non-sexual contact.

2. _____ The HIV positive patient may not exhibit any symptoms for as long as 10 years from coming into contact with the virus.

3. _____ The predominant abnormality in the HIV infection is the profound defect in normal immune functioning. This defect results in diminished body defenses and opportunistic infections that take advantage of the weakened system.

4. _____ A vaccine is available for HBV and is very strongly recommended for health care workers.

5. _____ The course of the HIV infection is predictable and similar from patient to patient.

6. _____ Hepatitis results in damage to the liver.

7. _____ It may take 6 weeks to six months following transmission of HIV for seroconversion (discovery of antibodies against HIV in the blood) to take place. It will take this long for the blood test to show positive.

8. _____ Women should know their HIV status before becoming pregnant.

9. List 3 behaviors that are considered to place a person at risk for contracting HIV.

   _____   _____

   _____

10. What do the initials AIDS stand for?

   _____

11. The name of the virus that causes AIDS is HIV. What does HIV stand for?

   _____

12. Name a type of cancer common in AIDS patients._____

13. What is the name of the common opportunistic lung problem that affects about 92% of AIDS patients?

   _____

14. Name 3 things that could be done to decrease the spread of HIV in the community.

   _____   _____

   _____

15. With proper techniques, health care workers are at minimal risk of contracting HIV. Name 2 specific exposure risks health care workers have.

   _____   _____

16. Name three symptoms an HIV infected patient may have in the early stages.

   _____

   _____

   _____

17. As part of good infection control measures, you should always protect yourself from coming in contact with body fluids.
   This is known as _____ precautions.

18. List one unique psycho-social problem an AIDS patient may have as compared to other terminally ill patients.

   _____

19. Describe 2 things you can do to avoid becoming infected with Hepatitis B.

   _____   _____

Chapter 10

Assisting with Personal Care

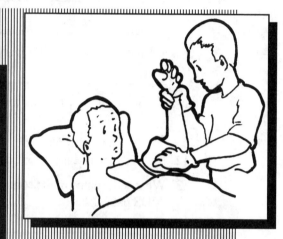

Learning Objectives

1. List at least 5 activities of daily living.

2. Describe what am and pm care consists of.

3. Explain what safety precautions need to be taken at bath and shower time.

4. Describe what special foot care precautions need to be taken for the diabetic resident and why.

5. Demonstrate the following procedures... bed bath, shower, tub bath, perineal care, back rub, and shampooing hair.

6. Describe denture care.

7. Explain what observations need to be made when bathing a resident.

8. Explain what oral care for the unconscious resident consists of.

9. Demonstrate how to assist the resident with oral care.

10. Document completed care for the resident on the flow sheet.

11. Demonstrate nail care, shaving, combing hair, and dressing residents.

Terms to Know

call signal
ADL's- activities of daily living
emesis basin
dentures
perineal (peri) care
am care
pm care
perineum
orange stick
wash mitt
emery board
oral hygiene
gangrene
decubitus ulcer
pressure area
necrosis
bedpan
commode
urinal
bony prominences
dental floss
dentures

These Are Four Steps You Must Take Before Starting Any Procedure

1. Wash your hands and use standard precautions including wearing gloves when appropriate.

2. Identify yourself to the resident and call them by name. Check their wrist band to establish identity.

3. Explain the procedure to the resident speaking clearly, slowly and directly while maintaining face to face contact whenever possible.

4. Provide privacy by closing doors, pulling privacy curtains, closing drapes or blinds.

End all procedures by doing the following...

1. Discard gloves if used.

2. Wash your hands.

3. Leave call signal within reach of resident.

4. Make sure that the resident is left in a safe and comfortable position.

Personal Care and Activities of Daily living

A resident comes to a long term care facility because they cannot take care of their own ADL's (Activities of Daily Living). You will be spending much of your work day taking care of the resident's ADL's. **Activities of daily living** are things a person does when they get up in the morning and that keeps them going throughout the day. This includes toileting, hygiene, bathing, dressing, oral care grooming and eating. Being clean and neat contributes to a person's comfort, sense of well-being and morale.

Residents all require A.M. and P.M. care.

A.M. care is given upon arising in the morning and getting ready for breakfast. It includes...

♦ bathroom, commode, bedpan or urinal use

♦ oral care (brushing teeth, or cleaning dentures, use of mouthwash, and flossing)

♦ washing face, hands, underarms

♦ brushing and caring for hair and nails and shaving male residents

♦ providing peri (perineal) care

- ♦ assisting resident to dress

- ♦ providing for bed bath, tub bath or shower as needed and/or according to schedule

P.M. care is given in the evening in preparation for sleep. It includes...

- ♦ bathroom, commode, bedpan or urinal use

- ♦ oral care (brushing teeth, or cleaning dentures, use of mouthwash and flossing)

- ♦ face, hands and underarms washing

- ♦ back rub

- ♦ perineal (peri) care

- ♦ dressing for bed

As in most procedures, encourage resident to do as much as they can for themselves. Some residents will need to have supplies set up for them, others need partial assistance, others need complete assistance. Check with your charge nurse and the resident care flow sheet as to the degree of assistance necessary for ADL's. If the resident is able to do part of ADL's, encourage and enable them to continue doing so. People derive a feeling of self worth in being as independent as possible. While the resident is completing their self care skills, work at straightening their unit or preparing their clothing and be available to assist them as needed.

Bathing

Bathing is important because it...

- ♦ gets rid of surface dirt and some microorganisms

- ♦ eliminates body odors

- ♦ stimulates circulation

- ♦ provides opportunity for observation of pressure areas, open areas, cuts, bruises, and rashes

There are different types of baths depending on the resident's condition and needs. The appropriate type is determined by the charge nurse, indicated on the flow sheet, and given by the nursing assistant. The different kinds of bathing are...

- ♦ complete bed bath- given to the resident who is not able to get out of bed and most likely, not able to help with the bathing process at all.

- ♦ partial bed bath- the resident is not able to get out of bed for the tub bath or shower and requires assistance. Encourage the resident to do as much as possible and assist with parts of the bath that they cannot do for themselves.

- ♦ whirlpool, Jacuzzi or tub bath - use great care in transferring the resident in and out and supervise for safety throughout the entire process.

- ♦ shower- the resident usually sits in a shower chair while taking a shower and may require partial or complete assistance. You are responsible for their safety at all times.

♦ waterless bathing – pre-packaged wash cloths that can be used in place of water and soap. They can be used at room temperature or put in the microwave for gentle warming. They are easy to use and less drying to the resident's skin.

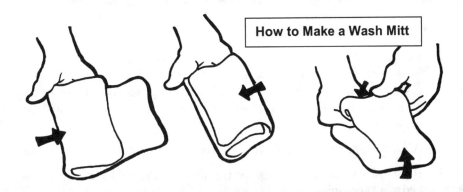

How to Make a Wash Mitt

Points to Remember About Bathing

1. Make sure to insure the resident's privacy. This means closing the door, pulling the curtain around the bed, pulling window blinds or curtains and only exposing the part of the body you are bathing at the time.

2. Bathing provides the best opportunity to observe skin condition, on the back, buttocks and over bony prominences. Report reddened, irritated, or open areas to the nurse.

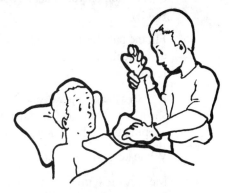

3. Encourage resident to do as much for themselves as possible.

4. Do not leave your resident unattended in the shower or bathroom. If they can do their own bathing, pull the curtain and stand on the other side of the curtain maintaining voice contact to insure resident safety.

5. Make sure to adequately rinse the resident and dry thoroughly. Soap that is not washed off can cause drying of skin.

6. Warm the lotion by putting the bottle of lotion in the basin of water. This will make it a more comfortable temperature when the lotion is applied.

7. Carefully plan ahead and get all your supplies ready.

8. During the bath, or when transporting the resident to the shower room, keep the resident covered with a bath blanket. This keeps them warm and protects their dignity and privacy.

9. Use disposable gloves when there is chance of direct contact with a body fluid. Use standard precautions.

10. Be respectful of the resident's preferences, fears and concerns regarding bathing. Remember that a resident does have the right to refuse a bath. Perhaps a partial bath or a different time for bathing would better accommodate the resident. Some confused residents may be fearful of bathing and need soothing reassurance and extra assistance. If a resident repeatedly refuses hygiene care, report this to your supervisor.

Procedure:

1. Prepare your supplies: soap, soap dish, wash cloth, wash basin, towels, bath blankets, lotion, **orange stick** (used to clean under nails), comb or brush, clean gown, clean linen, disposable gloves, linen bag or plastic laundry bag used for disposal of dirty basin. Stack clean linen on the chair in the resident's room in the order that you will use them. Apply disposable gloves.

2. Assist the resident with oral care as the need dictates, brushing teeth or doing denture care.

3. If the resident needs to use a bedpan or urinal do so at this point. Lower the head of the bed to a flat position.

4. Raise the bed height to a convenient height for you to maintain good body mechanics and avoid strain on your back. Lock the bed wheels in place. Keep side rails up as needed for safety.

5. Fill the bath basin 2/3 full. Use a bath thermometer to insure that the water temperature is no more than 105^0 F. Have the resident check the water temperature for their own comfort level.

6. Remove the bedspread and blanket off the bed, leaving the resident covered with a top sheet. Cover the top sheet with a bath blanket. Remove the top sheet from underneath keeping the bath blanket in place.

7. While keeping the resident covered with the bath blanket, remove the resident's gown.

8. Make a **wash mitt** as pictured. Wash from the cleanest part of the body to the dirtiest. This means you start by washing around the eyes. Wash from the part closest to the nose outward. Use another part of the washcloth for each eye to avoid cross contamination. Do not use soap around the eyes. Dry face using a blotting motion.

Bathe the resident in the following order...

1. Eyes
2. Face
3. Ears and neck
4. Arms and underarms
5. Chest
6. Abdomen
7. Feet and legs
8. Back and buttocks
9. Perineum

9. Cover the resident with a bath blanket. Wash, rinse and dry the ears and neck.

10. Support the elbow and extend the resident's arm. Move limbs gently avoiding force or over-extension of limbs. Wash, rinse and dry the shoulder, armpit (axilla) and arm. Do the same on the other arm. Wash, rinse and dry the hands. Do nail care as directed. (See page 160.)

11. Turn the bath blanket down to the waist. Wash the chest and also thoroughly dry under women's breasts. Be careful not leave any moisture under the breasts.

12. Place a towel over the chest. Pull bath blanket down to expose the abdominal area. Wash, rinse and dry the abdominal area. If the resident has folds of skin in the abdominal area be sure to carefully wash, rinse and thoroughly dry in the folds. Remove the towel and cover the resident with a bath blanket.

13. Remember to empty and change the bath water when it is dirty, cool to the touch or soapy. Remember to put the side rails up if you need to leave the bedside for even a few seconds if there is any risk that the resident could fall out of bed.

14. Move on to the lower extremities. Expose the leg furthest from you. Bend the knee and support the heel. Wash, rinse and dry. If the resident is capable of bending the leg, soak the foot in the basin. Wash, rinse and dry, including between each toe.

15. Check condition of toenails and skin on foot. Trim nails if you are allowed to do so (remember that the charge nurse or podiatrist needs to do nail care for the diabetic or anyone who has thick and difficult to trim nails). Report to the charge nurse any reddened, irritated or open areas. Repeat the process with the leg and foot closest to you.

16. Roll the resident away from you toward the raised siderail. Wash, rinse and dry the back. Give lotion rub to the back. Observe the skin especially over the **bony prominences** (areas where the bone is close to the skin surface). Report any reddened, irritated or open areas. Wash, rinse and dry the buttocks: apply lotion.

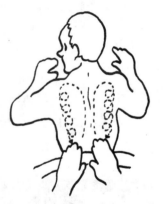

17. Water should be changed before giving perineal care. Do careful and thorough perineal care procedure as detailed on page 161.

18. Comb the resident's hair or have the resident comb their own hair if they are able.

19. Put clean gown or clean clothes on resident.

20. Position the resident comfortably with call light within easy reach. Lower the bed.

21. Empty, rinse and wipe wash basin and return to storage.

22. Discard gloves and wash your hands.

Partial Bed Bath

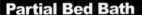

The equipment and procedure is the same as the complete bed bath, except that the resident may be able to do some of the bathing on their own. You can set up the equipment and supplies and hand them to the resident so they can do their own bathing. Assist or completely do the parts of the procedure they are not able to do. Most people feel good about being able to do for themselves and it also provides an excellent opportunity for joint and muscle movement.

Procedure:

1. Prepare your supplies and have them ready near the tub: bath thermometer, soap, wash cloths, wash basin, clean clothing, towels, shampoo, disposable gloves.

2. Make sure the tub is clean according to facility procedure.

3. Undress the resident in their room and put on robe and slippers. Make sure they are warm and covered for privacy. Transport them to the tub room either by ambulating them or by wheelchair.

4. Fill the tub half full. With bath thermometer make sure the temperature of the water does not exceed 105 F. Make sure it is comfortable for the resident.

5. To prevent slipping, put one towel on the bathtub edge for the resident to sit on and one inside the tub for the resident to stand on.

6. Assist the resident to get undressed and into the tub.

7. Assist with bathing if the resident needs it.

8. Shampoo the hair.

9. Put one towel on a chair.

10. Assist the resident out of the tub and onto the chair.

11. Dry the resident and dress them in their clean clothing.

12. Return the resident to their room.

13. Make the resident comfortable in the chair or in their bed if they are being transferred back to bed.

14. Leave call signal within reach of resident.

15. Clean and disinfect the tub according to facility procedure.

Showers

Many residents will take showers, either independently or with assistance. The care plan will indicate whether showering is the method of choice for the particular resident. There are several issues that deserve special attention...

♦ **Safety Precautions** are needed to prevent falling on wet, slippery surfaces in the shower room. Weak or unsteady residents need to use a shower chair. Shower chairs have wheels so residents can be transported and an open area on the plastic seat that allows water to run through. Handrails in the shower can also help steady a person in the shower. Never leave a resident alone in the shower room! Make sure non-skid shower mats are in place and used to prevent slipping. Check the water temperature by making sure that it does not exceed 105° and make sure it is comfortable for the resident.

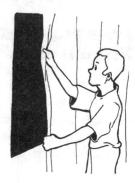

♦ **Privacy Needs** are crucial when undressing the resident, transporting them to and from the shower room and during the shower. Make sure the body is not unnecessarily exposed. Keep the resident covered for privacy and for comfort also.

Showering

Procedure:

1. Before starting gather your supplies and equipment: soap, 2 bath towels, 2 bath blankets, wash cloths, disposable gloves, deodorant, lotion, foot wear, clothing.

2. Make sure the shower room is clean and free of hazards. Make sure the rubber mat is in place. Check to make sure that the shower chair has been disinfected. Put out the "occupied" sign on the shower door. Toilet the resident before starting.

3. Pull the privacy curtain and prepare the resident for transfer to the shower room. Follow your particular facility procedure here. Some facilities will undress the resident in their room, wrap them in a bath blanket and then transport them to the shower room. Others will transport the resident to the shower room and undress them there.

4. If using a shower chair, lock the wheels for safety. If the resident is standing, encourage them to use the handrails to steady themselves.

5. Adjust the shower spray to a comfortable, gentle spray with temperature not exceeding 105° F.

6. Assist the resident with removing clothing or the bath blanket.

7. Put on disposable gloves and assist the resident as needed, cleaning from the cleanest part of the body to the dirtiest. Wash and rinse the perineal area last.

8. For residents who can safely stand alone, pull the curtain around them for privacy but stand immediately outside the curtain and maintain voice contact with them. **Do not** leave the shower room!

9. When the resident is finished, turn off the water flow and cover them with a bath blanket. Remove and discard your disposable gloves before leaving the shower room.

10. Use deodorant, powder or lotions as needed.

11. At some facilities the resident is dressed in the shower room and at other facilities they are wrapped in a bath blanket, transported back to their room where they are dressed.

12. Assist the resident as needed with the following: oral care, grooming, fingernail and toe nail care, and shaving. Use disposable gloves at any appropriate time.

13. Dispose of soiled laundry.

14. Change the resident's bed linen using gloves as necessary.

15. Assist the resident to a chair or back to bed if indicated.

16. Place the call light within reach of the resident and make sure they are comfortable.

17. Wash your hands before leaving the resident's room.

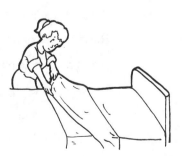

18. Return to the shower room and dispose of any used linens. Clean and disinfect the shower area and chair. Place the unoccupied sign on the door.

19. Document care provided and any observations made. Report to the nurse any reddened, irritated or open areas, or cuts, wounds or rashes observed.

Shampooing Hair

Shampooing can be done in the shower, bath tub, at the sink or in bed. Prevent soap or shampoo from getting into the resident's eyes. Massage the scalp well and rinse thoroughly. Bedridden residents need to have their hair shampooed while in bed. This can be done by use of no rinse shampoos, dry chemical shampoos or use of shampoo caps. Shampoo caps can be lightly warmed in the microwave for comfort, placed on the head and gently rubbed for 2-5 minutes depending on the length of the hair. The hair can then be towel dried and combed.

Combing the Hair

Procedure:

1. Place a towel over the resident's shoulders.

2. Comb the hair, one section at a time, being careful not to pull hard at the tangles.

3. Remove the towel from the shoulders.

4. Each resident should have a comb that is used only for them.

5. Remove towel from shoulders.

6. Observe and report to the charge nurse any sores or open areas on the scalp, scaly or excessive dandruff, or evidence of head lice.

Giving a Back Rub

A back rub can help the resident feel more comfortable, relax muscles, reduce tension and help stimulate circulation and reduce the possibility of skin breakdown. A backrub should be given as part of the bed bath, at bed time and for residents who spend much time in bed, when their position is changed.

Procedure:

1. Assemble equipment: towels, basin of water at 105^0 F., lotion.

2. Raise bed to comfortable working height.

3. Assist resident to turn on their side or on their abdomen.

4. Warm the lotion by putting the lotion container in a basin of water that is 105^0 F.

5. Warm your hands before applying a small amount of lotion into the palm of your hand. Rub your hands together to warm up the lotion.

6. Apply the lotion with long strokes up from the base of the spine to the shoulders and back of the neck, and downward in a circular motion.

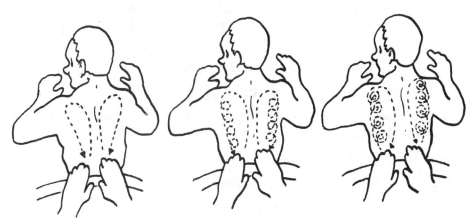

7. Continue this motion with gentle pressure for 2-3 minutes.

8. Observe skin condition and report to the nurse if necessary.

9. Close and retie the gown or dress the resident.

10. Assist the resident into a comfortable position.

11. Lower bed to a safe position for the resident and put curtain back to open position.

12. Place the call light within reach of the resident.

13. Wash your hands.

Applying Lotion Elsewhere on the Body

♦ When applying lotion to legs, merely pat it on gently. Do not massage it vigorously because it can cause complications regarding blood clots in the legs.

♦ Do not massage lotion near a pressure area since it can cause further tissue destruction.

Shaving the Resident

In order to maintain a clean shaven appearance and feel, shave the male resident daily. Some older women may need a shave on occasion also. Follow your facility policy regarding type of razor or shaver used. Some may use disposable safety razors, others may prefer electric razors.

Procedure:

1. Assemble your equipment at the bedside stand: electric razor, or safety blade razor, shaving brush, shaving cream, a basin of warm water (105° F), disposable gloves, washcloth, and face towel.

2. Put on disposable gloves.

3. Position the resident in a sitting position and spread a towel under the resident's chin.

4. Dampen a wash cloth with warm water and pat it against the resident's face to soften the resident's beard. Hold it in place for about 3 minutes.

5. If using a safety razor, lather up the shaving cream and apply to the face.

6. Using short, firm strokes and holding the skin taut, shave in the direction of hair growth. Shave downward from the sideburns down to the chin and then upwards from neck to chin. Make especially careful strokes under the nose and above the lips so as to not cut the resident.

7. Wash off shaving cream, pat the face dry.

8. If resident likes, apply lotion, or after shave.

9. Dispose of disposable razor, or clean the battery operated shaver. Carefully follow the disinfection procedure for the shaver.

10. Make the resident comfortable.

11. Leave the call within reach of the resident.

12. Discard disposable gloves and wash hands.

Oral Hygiene

Oral care includes brushing the teeth, mouth, gums and tongue of a resident who has teeth and flossing of teeth. For the resident without teeth, oral hygiene includes care of the dentures. Oral hygiene is important because it...

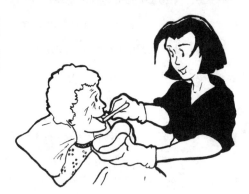

- ◆ Removes plaque off of teeth which maintains good dental and gum condition.

- ◆ Decreases bacteria in mouth which can cause infections

- ◆ Eliminates odors and bad taste in mouth thereby making foods taste better.

This also is an excellent time to observe and report to your charge nurse the following conditions...

> Dry or cracked lips
>
> Bleeding or swelling of gums
>
> White patches on mouth or tongue
>
> Redness, irritation or sores in mouth

Brushing Teeth

Teeth should be brushed every morning (before breakfast so the mouth and teeth feel fresh for breakfast), before going to bed and after meals. Many residents can do at least part of their oral care if the supplies are set up for them. Encourage the resident to do as much for themselves as possible. Some will need at least partial assistance and others will need total assistance.

Procedure

1. Assemble the following supplies: mouthwash, disposable cup, **emesis basin** (a kidney shaped pan), toothpaste, toothbrush, water, towel, dental floss, disposable gloves.

2. Roll the resident up in bed or position comfortably in chair. Cover the resident's chest with a towel.

3. Put on your disposable gloves.

4. Dilute the mouthwash with water and have the resident swish the mouthwash in their mouth and spit out into the basin.

5. Wet the toothbrush and put some toothpaste on it.

6. Brush the resident's teeth starting at one point in the mouth and working your way systematically around the mouth. Brush with a circular motion brushing along the gumline with each stroke. Brushing along the gumline helps avoid gum disease. Gently brush the tongue. Have the resident rinse with clean water and spit into the emesis basin close to their chin. Wipe the resident's mouth.

7. Once daily, use dental floss between each tooth. This is a very effective way to remove food particles between teeth.

8. Lubricate the resident's lips with petroleum jelly or other recommended lubricant.

9. Dispose of soiled linen.

10. Remove and discard your disposable gloves.

11. Lower the bed to a position safe to the resident.

12. Make sure the resident is comfortable.

13. Leave the call light within reach of the resident.

14. Put supplies and equipment away.

15. Wash your hands.

What About Oral Care for the Unconscious Resident?

The purpose of oral care for the unconscious resident is to reduce odor and infection in the mouth, remove plaque build up on the teeth and reduce drying of tissues of the mouth. An unconscious resident may have rapid, labored breathing, which dries the mouth, lips, and causes a thick coating on the tongue. **This resident requires oral care frequently, at least every two hours.**

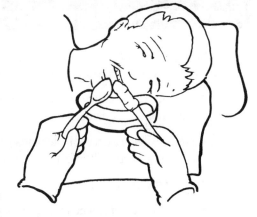

The unconscious resident cannot swallow, therefore great care needs to be exercised to prevent choking and aspiration (inhaling liquids into the lungs). To prevent aspiration, position the resident on his/her side with the head turned to one side over an emesis basin. Do not put fluids into the resident's mouth.

Oral Care for the Unconscious Resident

Procedure:

1. Assemble your supplies; emesis basin, disposable gloves, towel, commercially prepared swabs (lemon glycerin swabs or soft toothette), Vaseline jelly.

2. Remember that the unconscious resident may hear and understand you, so explain what you are about to do.

3. Put on your disposable gloves.

4. Roll up the head of the bed, position the resident in a side lying position with his/her head turned toward you.

5. Put the towel on the pillow under the resident's head and face. Put the emesis basin on the towel next to their mouth.

6. Gently open the mouth by using slight pressure on the cheek.

7. With a prepared swab or soft toothette, wipe the inside of the cheeks, roof of the mouth, tongue, teeth and along the gumline.

8. Discard the swabs or soft toothette into the emesis basin and continue with a fresh swab as necessary.

9. Examine the mouth, gums, lips, and tongue for redness, bleeding, sores, cracks, white patches or broken teeth. Report this to the charge nurse.

10. Dry the resident's face with a towel. Change any soiled linen or clothing.

11. Put a little bit of Vaseline jelly on the resident's lips.

12. Discard disposable gloves and equipment. Clean and put away the rest of the equipment.

13. Lower the position of the bed to a safe position and make sure the resident is comfortable.

14. Place the call light within easy reach of resident.

15. Wash your hands.

16. Document care and report observations to the charge nurse.

Dentures Require Special Care Too!

Dentures are artificial teeth. Denture care needs to be done in the morning upon arising and in the evening before going to bed. Some things to remember...

♦ Dentures are expensive to replace so take good care of them. Take precautions that they are not lost or damaged.

♦ Store dentures in cool, clean water in a labeled container. If they are left out open to the air they become brittle and susceptible to breaks. Hot water causes the denture to warp.

♦ Handle the dentures carefully to avoid dropping and possibly chipping or breaking them.

♦ Notify the nurse when the dentures do not fit properly, are chipped, cracked or missing.

♦ Make sure the resident has clean dentures in their mouth before eating.

Remember...

- ◆ Food can collect under the dentures so be sure to remove dentures and clean thoroughly.

- ◆ Loose or poorly fitting dentures can cause sores on the gums and inadequate chewing of food.

- ◆ Residents with dentures may have decreased awareness of how much to chew so may be more prone to choking. Cut up their food into bite size pieces if necessary.

- ◆ Some residents require adhesive paste for application of dentures for improved suction.

- ◆ Report to charge nurse any unusual observations made, such as any open or irritated areas in the mouth, inside cheeks or gums.

- ◆ Check for misplaced dentures in pockets of resident, on meal trays, or in bed linen.

Procedure:

1. Assemble equipment: emesis basin, toothpaste, towel, denture cup, gauze, mouthwash, and disposable gloves.

2. Cover the resident's chest with a towel.

3. Raise the head of the bed.

4. Put on your disposable gloves.

5. Line the emesis basin with tissues or paper towels. Ask resident to remove their dentures or assist them as necessary. If you need to remove the dentures for the resident, use a piece of gauze to grasp the slippery denture.

6. Take the emesis basin with the dentures to the sink.

7. To protect dentures from possible breakage, put a towel in the sink and fill the sink with water.

8. Rinse dentures in cool running water before brushing. Put toothpaste or denture cleanser on the toothbrush and brush the dentures thoroughly between teeth and underneath on the pink part of the denture. Hold the denture in the palm of your hand firmly. Rinse in cool, running water.

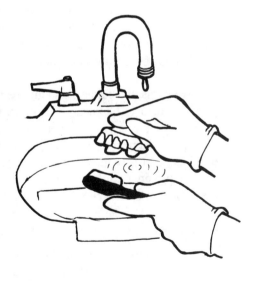

9. Rinse the denture cup, fill it with cool water or solution and put the dentures in the labeled cup. Store on bedside stand.

10. Have resident rinse mouth with half mouthwash, half water solution.

11. Check the mouth, lips, and gums for any reddened, irritated, or open areas and report to the nurse.

12. Dispose of sink liner in appropriate container and drain sink. Remove, discard disposable gloves, towels and supplies. Clean and store the rest of equipment.

13. Make the resident comfortable, roll down head of bed.

14. Leave the call light within easy reach of resident.

15. Wash your hands.

16. Document the care provided.

To remove dentures...

Place your thumb inside toward the roof of the mouth and two fingers on outside. Take them out of the mouth one side at a time. Use gentle rocking motion and outward pulling motion to remove them.

Perineal Care (Peri-care)

Perineal care means cleaning the external genitalia and the rectal area. It needs to be done during am & pm care, during the shower or bath, and after each episode of incontinence and diarrhea stool. If possible the resident should do their own peri care. They may need assistance in assembling supplies or they may need partial or full assistance, depending on their limitations.

Perineal care is important for your residents because it...

♦ restores and maintains comfort for the incontinent person.

♦ removes surface microorganisms

♦ eliminates odor.

♦ prevents skin irritation and infections.

The perineum is a warm, moist area. It is moist because there are sweat glands and mucous secretions in this area. Additionally this is a semi-enclosed area since it is between the thighs, with close fitting underwear surrounding the area. This is a warm, moist environment ideal for bacteria growth, unpleasant odors, infections and skin irritation.

To prevent this, the perineum should be washed daily with soap and water, thoroughly rinsed and dried. Remember that soap can be drying to the skin and if not rinsed off well can cause skin itchiness. Some facilities prefer use of a special peri solution instead. Bowel and stool contain bacteria. If there is prolonged contact with stool (feces) and the urethra and vagina, this can contribute to urinary tract infections (UTI's). This is especially a problem in the female because of the close proximity of the rectum to the exterior urinary opening. **It is particularly important to wipe from front to back when wiping after BM's and when doing peri-care.**

Procedure:

1. Assemble equipment: disposable gloves, toilet paper, disposable bed protectors, bedpan and cover, wash cloth, peri-care solution.

2. Raise the bed to a comfortable working height for you.

3. Place a waterproof bed protector under the resident's buttocks.

4. While maintaining privacy, cover the resident with the bath blanket and remove the top sheet from underneath. Expose the perineum only.

5. Put on disposable gloves.

6. Have the resident lie on their back with their knees flexed and separated.

7. The **perineum in the male** means the penis, scrotum, rectal area. Peri-care for the male means cleaning the penis from the urethral opening at the tip toward the bottom of the penis and scrotum and the rectal area. In the uncircumcised male: gently retract the foreskin, cleanse the penis and replace the foreskin. Wash the scrotum and finally around the rectal area. Dry the genitalia gently.

8. The **perineum in the female** means the pubic area, outer urethral opening, outer vaginal opening, labia and rectal area. Spray the perineum with peri-solution or apply soap to the washcloth according to facility procedure. Separate labia during washing. Cleanse from front to back. In the female it is essential to **wipe from front to back** and change location on the wash cloth with each wipe. Do not wipe back and forth! This helps prevent introduction of microorganisms from around the rectum to the urethra, a contributing cause of urinary tract infections (UTI's).

9. In both male and female, wash entire perineal area with soapy washcloth moving from front to back, using clean area on wash cloth with each stroke. Rinse the entire area in this same manner. Dry the perineum with a towel using a blotting motion.

10. Turn the resident on his/her side. Cleanse the rectal area without contaminating the perineal area.

11. Observe for any reddened open or irritated area in the perineum and the rectal area, or unusual odors or discharge and report to the charge nurse.

12. Remove bedpan, bed protector, or wet incontinent pad. Place a clean, dry pad under the resident.

13. Cover the resident with a top sheet and remove bath blanket from underneath.

14. Lower the bed to a safe height for the resident and reposition the resident.

15. Dispose of soiled linen.

16. Empty, rinse, and wipe basin and return to proper storage. Follow facility policy regarding disinfection of equipment.

17. Remove and dispose gloves without contaminating self after returning basin to storage.

18. Place the call light within resident's reach.

19. Wash hands.

Dressing

Dressing oneself can be excellent exercise. Encourage the residents to do as much for themselves as they are able, assist with what they cannot do. Some residents may have difficulty with such things as zipping up their pants or clothing up the back, putting on their shoes, tying their shoes, or buttoning buttons. You may need to help with these tasks. Residents may be evaluated by an occupational therapist who may make recommendations regarding some dressing assistive devices that could help residents help themselves. This can include button hookers that are helpful in buttoning buttons and long shoe horns to help put on slip on shoes. There are specially designed clothes that are helpful also, such as shoes or clothes with velcro closures, clothes that open in the front for easy dressing and undressing.

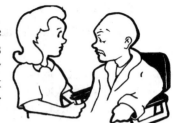

Dressing can also provide an opportunity for choices for the resident in what to wear. Ask residents what their preferences are. For the confused resident you can assist in the process by bringing in options to the resident. For example you can ask "would you like to wear this blue dress, this pink floral dress or the green striped dress?"

A resident who may have a weak or paralyzed arm or leg will need to have that limb put into the sleeve or pant leg first. When undressing, remove clothing from the non-paralyzed side first and then the weak side.

Always make sure the clothing is neat, clean and in good repair. Any torn clothing should be given to the charge nurse who will either arrange repair or arrange for any additional clothing needed. Soiled clothing should be put into soiled laundry hamper. Dress resident in as attractive a manner as possible. If you notice that the resident is running low on clothing items, talk to your charge nurse. Make sure the resident is dressed warmly enough in street clothing. Check the name tags to make sure that the clothing belongs to the resident.

Dressing a Resident with an Affected Arm

(An affected arm may be one that is paralyzed or unable to move normally for any other reason.)

Procedure:

1. Provide for privacy for the resident during the procedure.

2. Offer the resident a choice of what clothing they would like to wear.

3. Remove the resident's clothing without completely exposing the resident.

4. Assist the resident to put their affected arm through the sleeve first before putting the unaffected arm through the other sleeve.

5. While dressing the resident, move their body gently, avoiding force and over-extension of joints.

6. Assist resident with the lower extremity dressing. Put on non-skid footwear. Make sure the bed is lowered to a safe height before standing the resident.

7. Make sure the resident is dressed appropriately and seated.

8. Place soiled clothing in soiled laundry.

9. Leave call light within reach of the resident.

Hand and Fingernail Care

Procedure:

1. Follow your facility policy regarding whether you are allowed to clip and clean nails for your resident.

2. Assemble equipment: basin, soap, towel and wash cloth, bath thermometer, lotion, nail clippers, emery board, orange stick.

3. Explain the procedure to the resident.

4. Sit the resident in a comfortable position.

5. Fill a basin of water with warm water and use a bath thermometer to make sure the temperature is about 105° F. Put the basin on the overbed table.

6. Have the resident soak their hands in the basin of water for about 5 minutes and then wash their hands.

7. Gently clean under each fingernail with an orange wood stick. Wipe the orange wood stick on a towel after each nail. Check with the charge nurse before using orange wood stick on a diabetic resident. Dry the hands with a towel.

8. Use nail clippers to cut the nails straight across.

9. Use an emery board to smooth the nails and round the edges.

10. Apply lotion onto the resident's hands.

11. Empty the water from the basin. Follow your facility policy regarding cleaning and storing equipment.

12. Wash your hands.

13. Leave signaling device within reach of the resident.

Foot Care

Procedure:

1. Gather equipment and supplies at the bedside: basin, water bath thermometer, soap, towels, wash cloth, lotion, gloves (if there is a risk of contacting body fluids), orange wood sticks.

2. Provide for privacy and explain procedure to the resident.

3. Apply gloves if there is a possibility of contacting body fluids.

4. Position the resident in a comfortable sitting position.

5. Place towel on the floor in front of the resident and put the basin of water on the towel.

6. Check the water temperature with a bath thermometer. It should be about 105° F.

7. Submerge the feet into the basin and allow feet to soak about 10 minutes.

8. Wash the feet using a wash cloth, soap and water.

9. Wash, rinse and dry between each toe.

10. If you will be trimming the toe nails, use a nail clipper and cut straight across and file the edges gently. Do not trim the nails too short and be careful not to nick or cut surrounding tissue. Before trimming nails, check with your charge nurse to be sure that you are allowed to do so.

11. Clean underneath each nail with an orange wood stick and wipe the orange wood stick on the towel after each nail.

12. Apply lotion to the feet but not between the toes.

13. Report any reddened, irritated, open areas or any corns or calluses to your charge nurse.

14. Assist the resident with putting on clean socks and shoes.

15. Assist the resident to a comfortable position and leave signaling device within easy reach.

16. Empty the water from the basin. Follow your facility policy regarding cleaning and storing equipment.

17. Wash your hands.

Special Considerations

Foot and toe nail care is a special need that resident's have. It frequently is one of the first ADL's that residents can no longer do for themselves. Doing one's own foot care requires a certain amount of flexibility in having to bend down to reach one's feet and toes, it requires good vision and dexterity in handling nail clippers. Residents frequently require partial or complete assistance with foot and nail care.

1. Assess the resident's foot condition daily and report problem areas to the charge nurse. Things to watch for are...

> One or both feet cold to the touch
>
> Red, pale or cyanotic (bluish discoloration) areas
>
> Complaints of pain
>
> Open or irritated areas
>
> Corns, calluses, or bunions
>
> Thick or broken nails
>
> Hang nails or ingrown toenails
>
> Bruises
>
> Edema

2. Provide foot care daily. This includes washing feet, drying carefully between each toe, and applying lubricating lotion. Do not apply lotion between toes.

3. Trim nails only if directed to do so. Do not trim nails of diabetic residents, or those with circulation problems. Any cut to the skin during this procedure could result in slow healing of cuts or the possibility of the cut never healing and leading to infection, gangrene, and possibly amputation. For diabetics or residents with circulatory problems, nail trimming should only be done by a podiatrist or the charge nurse.

Special Foot Care Needs

People with poor circulation due to congestive heart failure or diabetes are susceptible to serious complications. Sluggish circulation does not adequately nourish the tissues in the extremities, particularly the feet. This person is susceptible to infections and slow healing cuts, wounds or sores. This can lead to **gangrene** and possibly death. Gangrene may result in an amputation of a limb in an effort to save a persons life. 40-50% of amputations occur to the diabetic resident. Residents with poor circulation and/or the diabetic resident require a special regime of foot care:

1. Do not trim the toe nails of the diabetic resident. This should be done by the podiatrist or licensed nurse. This is also true for any resident who has very thick nails or otherwise difficult to handle nails.

2. Feet should be bathed in lukewarm water daily and rinsed thoroughly. Carefully and gently pat the feet dry with a soft towel. Do not apply lotion between the toes since this may increase the chance of fungus growth between the toes. Dry between each toe.

3. The resident should wear clean socks that are changed daily.

4. Shoes should fit well but not tight. Shoes should be changed daily, allowing the worn pair of shoes to air out.

5. New shoes should be "broken in" gradually.

6. Notify your charge nurse immediately if you notice any reddened, irritated, or open areas on the resident's feet, or any reddened or "hot" area on the resident's legs.

7. Examine the condition of your resident's feet daily. Remember the resident may have no sensation or feeling in their extremities so may not complain of any problem.

8. Avoid any extremes of temperature to the resident's feet.

9. Avoid anything tight around the resident's legs or ankles that might in any way reduce the blood supply to the feet.

10. Be aware that smoking reduces circulation to the feet.

Applying lotion to dry skin on resident's heel

Procedure:

1. Put lotion in your hands and rub them together to warm the lotion.

2. Raise and support the foot.

3. Apply the lotion to the heel in a circular motion.

4. Lower the foot.

5. Cover the foot or put on sock or stocking.

6. Wash your hands.

Skin

Skin covers most of the body and is our largest organ. It is the first line of defense against infection. Skin produces an oil that keeps it moist and soft. Blood vessels in the skin keep the internal body temperature warm, and the sweat glands in the skin help the body get rid of water and salt through perspiration. Nerves and nerve endings in the skin let the skin feel the outside world by touch, temperature change, pressure and pain.

There are three main layers in both young and aging skin. However, normal, aging skin is very different from young skin.

How the Aging Process Affects the Three Layers of Skin

♦ The EPIDERMIS, or outer layer, gradually gets thinner during aging. This makes it easier for skin to break down. If the skin becomes waterlogged from incontinence, it may become swollen and macerated which may lead to skin injury.

♦ The DERMIS, or middle layer, flattens with aging. This affects the nerves and nerve endings so that the skin is less sensitive to touch, temperature change, pressure and pain. Rubbing or damage from urine wetness can cause this layer to pull away from the epidermis which can lead to skin breakdown.

♦ The SUBCUTANEOUS, or fatty layer, gets thinner with age. This makes skin less able to absorb injury and more sensitive to cold.

Decubitus Prevention

Skin at Risk Sites

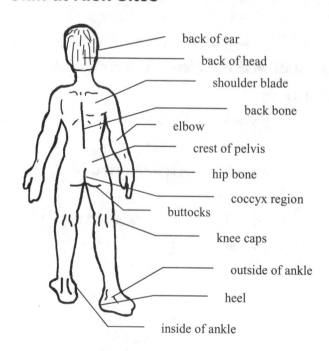

Pressure Areas

Lack of good care in nursing will cause a breakdown of tissue in these areas.

8 hours of neglect will take 1 to 5 weeks to heal.

back of ear
back of head
shoulder blade
back bone
elbow
crest of pelvis
hip bone
coccyx region
buttocks
knee caps
outside of ankle
heel
inside of ankle

What is a Decubitus Ulcer?

Understanding how decubitus ulcers or pressure ulcers develop is key to their prevention. Deep ulcers are caused by the compression of soft tissue between bony prominences and an external surface such as a chair or bed. **Bony prominences** are areas where the bones come close to the surface of the skin such as coccyx (tail-bone), hip, heel, elbow, etc. When a resident remains in one position for too long, the pressure obstructs blood flow, causing ischemia. Ischemia means lack of oxygen and nutrients to an area. This can lead to necrosis or death of tissue. Underlying tissue damage can occur before there is an visible surface damage. This means caregivers need to always be vigilant and not wait to see visible symptoms of damage before careful nursing care is started.

Decubitus ulcers or pressures ulcers can be a devastating problem for residents. Once one develops it can take up to a year or longer to heal. In a worse case scenario the ulcer can become infected, and may even lead to septicemia (a body wide infection) and death. Obviously prevention is crucial.

Residents Susceptible to Skin Breakdowns...

- incontinent residents

- obese residents

- thin residents

- decreased mobility residents

- diabetic residents

- poor circulation residents

- malnourished or anemic residents

- dehydrated residents

- residents in a cast

- residents with spasticity/rigidity and contractures

- residents with skin changes such as decrease in elasticity and subcutaneous fat

- residents with dementia and decreased level of consciousness and/or coma

Causes of Pressure Sores

Pressure - resulting in decreased blood flow to the skin causing edema, hypoxia (lack of oxygen) and eventual necrosis (death of tissue). Pressure occurs from resident sitting or lying in one position for too long. How long is too long depends on the particular patient, but this time should not exceed two hours!

Friction - skin rubbing against resistive surface such as a bed sheet. This damage can occur if the resident is dragged over the bed linen. It can rub off the top layer of skin or cause superficial irritation.

Moisture - urinary incontinence fecal soilage and/ or perspiration drastically increase the risk of pressure sore formation. Waterlogged skin is more vulnerable to both friction and pressure because the excessive moisture weakens the cell walls. When exposed to the pressure, waterlogged cells rupture easily.

Shearing Forces - this causes deep tissue damage. If the resident's head of bed is elevated 30 degrees or more, they tend to slide down. The skin tends to stick to the sheets and it pulls away from the underlying tissue. In the process, arteries stretch and tear, reducing blood flow to the area. The sacrum/coccyx area is frequently affected by shearing forces resulting in a decubitus.

Skin Injury - any break in skin integrity.

Nursing Prevention of Pressure Sores

Prevent Pressure

- Mattress: water, alternating air pressure, floatation, etc.

- Positioning and rotation at least every two hours, use of appropriate support pillows and cushions to redistribute pressure. In wheelchair use of cushions and positioning devices.

- Bed cradle or frame that protrudes above the mattress and prevents the top linen from touching the resident's feet and legs.

- Maintain good body alignment by keeping hips and bones flexed. To achieve this, support the resident's back with a pillow and put a pillow between the knees.

- While the resident is supine, do not have their heels touching the mattress. Suspend the heels by placing a pillow under the lower legs or use heel protectors.

- A resident who is seated should shift weight every 15 minutes.

Prevent Friction

- Lubrication with skin care lotion and/or application of incontinent spray.

- Avoid dragging of resident in bed. Use a draw sheet and move the resident up in bed with help from another nursing assistant.

- Avoid wrinkles in sheets.

- Do not massage reddened areas over bony prominences since this can cause further damage.

Prevent Shearing

- Keep head of bed flat or not more than 30^0

- Use of sheepskin or heel/elbow protectors

Control Moisture

- Incontinence management: frequent change of underpads, etc.

- Scheduled toileting or bowel and bladder training, and use of absorbent pads.

- Skin cleansing

Avoid Skin Injury

- ◆ Avoid particles in bed.

- ◆ Staff to avoid wearing jewelry that may scratch the resident.

- ◆ Staff and resident to have clean, trimmed fingernails.

Additionally...

Maintain good nutrition and good fluid intake (2500 cc. daily) for the resident. A high protein diet helps healing.

Stages of Pressure Sores:

Stage 1 Ulcer: Skin is intact (not broken), may appear dark red or mottled (blotchy), feel hard or warm. Upon position change, you may notice that redness over a bony prominence does not disappear for up to 30 minutes. Good skin care can halt progression through the following stages and development of a decubitus ulcer can be avoided.

Stage 2 Ulcer: The skin becomes broken, cracked, possibly blistered or appears as a shallow crater. The surrounding area may become reddened. It can involve the epidermis, dermis or both.

Stage 3 Ulcer: Skin break with deep tissue involvement and exposure of subcutaneous tissue. The ulcer may or may not be infected. The ulcer or hole penetrates all the way down to just above the muscle tissue. The ulcer is black around the edges due to tissue death (necrosis). The nerves are now dead so it is not painful at this stage. It will take months to heal.

Stage 4 Ulcer: Extensive ulceration with penetration to the muscle, tendon or bone with tissue necrosis. The ulcer may become infected, possibly with staphylococcus aureus and if not treated aggressively may become deadly.

Chapter 10 - Quiz Yourself

True or False

1. _____ Dentures can be wrapped in a tissue and stored in a drawer.

2. _____ Oral care for an unconscious resident should be done once every shift.

3. _____ When bathing the resident, start with the area around the eyes first.

4. _____ When dressing a resident who has a paralyzed right arm, put the left hand in the sleeve first.

5. _____ You should carefully trim the nails of a diabetic resident.

6. _____ Bathing provides the best opportunity for observation of skin condition.

7. _____ When trimming nails, cut straight across and file the edges with an emery board.

8. _____ Our first line of defense against infection is skin.

9. _____ There are significant changes in skin as a person ages, making them more susceptible to skin breakdown.

10. _____ A resident who is dehydrated is more prone to development of a decubitus ulcer.

Choose one correct answer

11. When giving a resident a bed bath, the resident should be covered and only the part of the body being bathed should be exposed. This is because...

   a. we need to provide privacy
   b. we need to keep the resident warm
   c. all of the above
   d. none of the above

Answer the following

12. Name two possible causes of skin breakdowns.

   _____

   _____

13. Describe two specific things you can do to help prevent skin breakdowns.

   _____

   _____

Chapter 11

Vital Signs

Learning Objectives

1. Define vital signs and what they tell us about a persons medical condition.

2. List sites where a body temperature can be measured, why each site would be utilized and normal values for each.

3. Demonstrate the proper procedure for obtaining temperature using electronic, tympanic and glass non-mercury thermometers.

4. Define pulse and take a radial pulse accurately.

5. Measure a blood pressure accurately.

6. Explain systolic and diastolic blood pressure.

7. Document vital sign results on a flow sheet.

8. Explain what normal values are for temperature, pulse, respirations, and blood pressure.

9. List at least 4 pulse points in the body and a description of where they are.

10. Describe three characteristics you look for when checking a pulse.

11. Count respirations accurately.

Terms to Know

calibrated
vital signs
temperature
respiration
pulse
blood pressure
oral temperature
axillary temperature
tympanic temperature
rectal temperature
glass non-mercury thermometer
electronic thermometer
carotid pulse
brachial pulse
radial pulse
apical pulse
stethoscope
sphygmomanometer
systolic blood pressure
diastolic blood pressure
hypotension
hypertension
respirations
Fahrenheit
Centigrade
diaphragm of stethoscope
febrile
tachycardia
bradycardia
dyspnea

Vital Signs

One of the very important tasks a nursing assistant has to do is taking vital signs.

Vital signs are...

Temperature (T)

Pulse (P)

Respiration (R)

Blood pressure (BP)

Vital signs are exactly that; signs that are vital to life and condition of the resident. They indicate very important functions of the body. They may indicate a crucial, perhaps even life threatening change in the resident.

It is essential that nursing assistants know how to accurately take vital signs, know what the normal values are and promptly report to the charge nurse any abnormalities. You may be the first person to identify an abnormal vital sign value. It is important that you notify the charge nurse promptly so that further appropriate action can be taken. An example may be a resident who has an elevated temperature. This may indicate an inflammation or infection which needs prompt treatment. The first step is the nursing assistant recognizing the elevated temperature and notifying the charge nurse. The charge nurse then will examine the resident, assess the situation, notify the physician who may make a diagnosis and possibly prescribe treatment. Another example may be a resident with a significantly elevated blood pressure. If this remains unnoticed the resident may have a stroke with either severe disabilities or possibly even death. If the nursing assistant identifies the elevated blood pressure and reports it to the charge nurse, prompt treatment may be started to bring down the blood pressure to within normal limits, thus avoiding stroke and disabilities or death.

Being accurate is very important. If you are unsure of your measurement, check with your supervisor. Your resident's life and welfare are at stake!

Temperature

Definition: **Temperature** is a measure of heat in the body. Body temperature can be lower in the morning and higher in the evening. Younger people normally have higher body temperature than older people. A person with an elevated body temperature is said to be **febrile**.

Elevated temperature may indicate...

Infection

Inflammatory process

Dehydration

Extremely warm environment

Low body temperature may indicate...

Shock

Hypothermia

Reaction to some medications

In the United States we generally use the Fahrenheit scale for the measurement of temperature. The **Fahrenheit** thermometer has temperature ranging from 96° F to 106° F. The abbreviation for Fahrenheit is F. The freezing point on the Fahrenheit scale is 32° and boiling is 212° F.

Most of the world outside of the United States uses the **Centigrade**, also called Celsius measurement of temperature. The abbreviation for Centigrade is C. The freezing point on the centigrade scale is 0° and boiling is 100° C.

Ways to Take a Temperature

Temperatures can be taken in several different places. Different locations may be preferable under certain conditions. It is important for you to understand what the locations are, what the normal values are and which route is preferable for which resident. The different routes are...

> tympanic - in the ear
>
> axillary(ax) - in the armpit
>
> rectal(R) - in the rectum
>
> oral - in the mouth
>
> temporal artery – forehead

Normal Body Temperatures

Location	Average		Normal Range	
Oral	98.6° F	(37° C)	97.6° to 99.6° F	(36.5° to 37.5° C)
Rectal	99.6° F	(37.5° C)	98.6° to 100.6° F	(37° to 38.1° C)
Axillary	97.6° F	(36.5° C)	96.6° to 98.6° F	(35.9° to 37° C)
Tympanic	98.6° F	(37° C)	98.6° F	(37° C)
Temporal	99.6° F	(37.5° C)	99.6° F	(37.5° C)

Types of Thermometers

The **electronic thermometer** is a battery operated thermometer that registers a persons temperature on the lighted display. The electronic thermometer registers within seconds, usually under a minute. The result is displayed digitally. For hygienic purposes a plastic sheath is used to cover the probe and discarded after use. This is a quick, safe and accurate method. Rectal probes are colored red and oral probes are colored blue.

Tympanic or Aural Thermometer

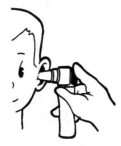

This electronic thermometer can be the fastest and most accurate way to take a temperature. An instrument is inserted into the outer ear canal and the results are printed digitally. The temperature registers within 1-3 seconds and it can be used under most circumstances. If a person has lots of ear wax, this method will not work. Do not do a tympanic temperature if the resident has an ear disorder or has ear drainage.

Measuring Tympanic Temperature Procedure

1. Assemble your equipment: tympanic thermometer, disposable probe cover, pen, paper.

2. Apply the disposable probe cover to the thermometer.

3. Gently lift the top of the outer ear so it straightens the ear canal.

4. Gently slide the thermometer in as far as it will go.

5. Hold the handle as pictured.

6. Push the scan button. Hold the thermometer until the temperature flashes on the display.

7. Record the results (the thermometer can be set in either rectal or oral equivalents)

8. Wash your hands.

Temporal Artery Thermometer

Temperature can be measured at the temporal artery in the forehead. This is quick and easy and registers in 3 to 4 seconds. Simply slide the thermometer across the forehead. Follow manufacturers directions regarding use, cleaning and storing.

Temperature Sensitive Tape

The thermometer is applied to the forehead or abdomen. It changes color in 15 seconds to indicate the temperature.

Disposable Oral Thermometer

A thermometer is place in the mouth for 60 seconds. Colored dots indicate the temperature.

Glass Non-mercury Thermometer

A series of long and short lines indicate the temperature. The non-mercury thermometer has replaced the mercury thermometer because we have become increasingly aware that mercury is a hazardous material. You may still find mercury thermometers in homes. If the glass mercury thermometer should break, do not touch the mercury and treat it as a hazardous waste. A disposable plastic sheath is used for hygienic purposes. Special precautions are used when using a glass thermometer.

1. Make sure the thermometer is not chipped or cracked.

2. Shake down the thermometer firmly with strong downward thrusts. Make sure you are away from any hard objects that you could accidentally strike the thermometer on.

3. Stay with the resident the entire time the thermometer is in place.

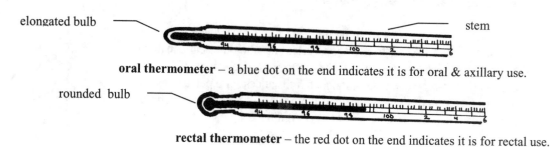

elongated bulb   stem

oral thermometer – a blue dot on the end indicates it is for oral & axillary use.

rounded bulb

rectal thermometer – the red dot on the end indicates it is for rectal use.

Oral Temperature

A **glass thermometer** is inserted under the tongue and should be maintained in place for at least 3 minutes with lips sealed. An **electronic oral thermometer** can register in several seconds. In order to have an accurate reading, the resident should not have had anything hot or cold to drink, nor smoked a cigarette within 20 minutes prior to the temperature being taken. Do NOT take the resident's temperature orally if...

♦ they are unconscious

♦ they have history of seizures

♦ they have an oxygen mask over the face or receive oxygen by nasal canula

♦ the person is confused, restless, delirious or under the age of 6.

♦ they cannot keep their lips sealed

♦ they cannot safely hold the thermometer in place.

♦ they are sneezing or coughing.

♦ they have partial paralysis of the face.

Measuring Oral Temperature

Procedure:

1. Assemble your equipment: gloves, oral thermometer, tissues, something to write with, pad of paper, watch, and a container for used thermometers.

2. Rinse the thermometer that was soaking in disinfection solution and wipe it off with tissues.

3. Hold the thermometer by the stem firmly and make firm downward thrusts to shake the mercury down to 96° F or lower.

4. Wear gloves due to the possibility of exposure to blood, body fluids, mucous membranes, or excretions.

5. Gently insert the bulb end of the thermometer under the tongue of the resident and to one side. Ask the resident to close lips around the thermometer.

6. Stay with the resident while the thermometer remains in place for 3 minutes.

7. While grasping the stem end, remove the thermometer. Remove and discard the sheath. Read the thermometer.

8. Shake the thermometer down to 96° F or lower. Clean the thermometer and/or return it to the container used for thermometers.

9. Place the signaling device within reach of the resident.

10. Remove gloves and wash your hands.

11. Record the temperature reading.

12. Follow the facility procedure for disinfection of thermometers.

Rectal Temperature

The **glass non-mercury thermometer** is inserted into the rectum and should be held in place for 3-5 minutes. An **electronic rectal thermometer** can take several seconds.

Do not take the temperature rectally if the resident has had...

- ◆ rectal surgery recently, such as hemorrhoid surgery

- ◆ rectal surgery which closed the rectum, such as a resident who has a colostomy or ileostomy

- ◆ diarrhea

Measuring Rectal Temperature

Procedure:

1. Assemble your equipment: rectal thermometer, lubricating jelly, disposable gloves, something to write with, pad of paper, watch.

2. Put on disposable gloves. Pull curtain and provide privacy.

3. Rinse thermometer that was soaking in disinfection solution and wipe it off with tissues.

4. Shake the thermometer down.

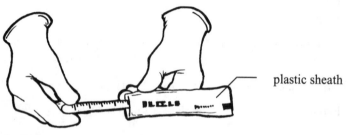

plastic sheath

5. Apply a plastic sheath over the thermometer

6. Lubricate the bulb end of the thermometer with the lubricant.

7. Position the resident on their side with the upper leg bent.

8. Expose only the buttocks, keep resident covered elsewhere.

9. Insert the thermometer 1-1/4 inches into the anus. Never force the thermometer. Hold onto the thermometer the entire 3 minutes.

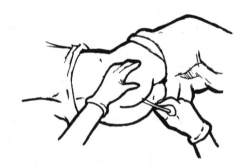

10. Remove the thermometer. Remove and dispose the plastic sheath.

11. Read and record the temperature.

12. Shake the thermometer down to 96° F or lower.

13. Rinse the thermometer in cold, soapy water. Place it in the disinfectant solution.

14. Remove and dispose of the disposable gloves. Wash your hands.

15. Place the resident in a comfortable and safe position.

16. Leave the signaling device within reach of the resident.

Axillary Temperature

The oral thermometer is placed in the armpit (axilla). This is the least accurate method and is rarely used. Place the thermometer in the center of the axilla. The resident needs to firmly cross his/her arm over the chest, holding the thermometer in place for 10 minutes.

How to read a glass thermometer

Procedure:

1. Hold the thermometer at the stem end, not the bulb end.

2. Hold the thermometer at your eye level.

3. Look above the numbers but below the lines. Rotate the thermometer until you can see the silver line extending from the bulb end.

4. Find the nearest degree (the long line) immediately below where the silver line ends. This tells you the degree. Now count how many two-tenths of a degree (the short lines) are above the degree. This gives you the complete temperature. Remember that the two tenths of a degree are counted in even numbers such as .2, .4, .6, .8, never .1,.3.,.5, .7, .9.

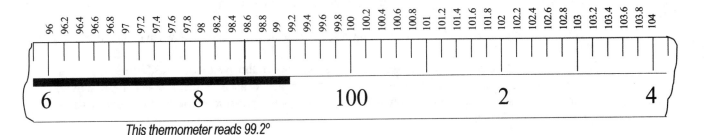

This thermometer reads 99.2°

Fahrenheit Scale

long lines = 1 degree   short lines = .2 degrees   (count by .2 .4 .6 . 8)

Read These Thermometers

Write temperatures here

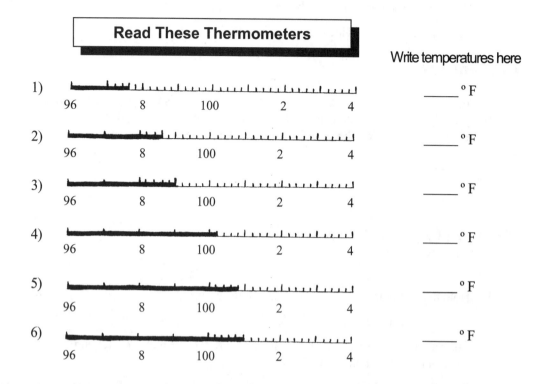

1) _____ ° F

96   8   100   2   4

2) _____ ° F

96   8   100   2   4

3) _____ ° F

96   8   100   2   4

4) _____ ° F

96   8   100   2   4

5) _____ ° F

96   8   100   2   4

6) _____ ° F

96   8   100   2   4

Blood Pressure

Definition: **Blood pressure** is the measurement of the force of the blood against artery walls.

The **systolic pressure** is the pressure in the artery when the heart contracts.

The **diastolic pressure** is the pressure in the artery when the heart relaxes between contractions.

High blood pressure (hypertension) affects about 50 million Americans. There is a clear relationship between untreated hypertension and a greater chance of heart attack, heart failure, stroke and kidney disease. It is important to monitor blood pressure regularly to insure that it is within normal limits.

In 2003 the American Heart Association issued new guidelines for desirable blood pressure. A new classification of "prehypertension" was added. People in this range are at higher risk of complications and more likely to develop high blood pressure where medication is required. The desire is to motivate people in this category to adopt healthier life styles before they develop hypertension.

New blood pressure guidelines

Blood pressure (mm Hg)	Optimal	Prehypertension	Hypertension
Systolic (top number)	Less than 120	120-139	140 or higher
Diastolic (bottom number)	Less than 80	80-89	90 or higher

Taking a blood pressure

When taking the blood pressure, the first sound you hear is the systolic. The heart beat sound will continue, when it stops this is the diastolic pressure. The numbers are measured as millimeters of mercury. The abbreviation indicating this is mm.Hg.

An example of how blood pressure is written is... $\dfrac{120}{80}$ The top number is systolic.
The bottom number is diastolic.

Hypotension means a low blood pressure. **Hypertension** means an elevated blood pressure.

Before Starting

The blood pressure is measured by using a **sphygmomanometer** or **blood pressure cuff**.

- Allow resident to relax about 15 minutes before taking blood pressure.

- Select the correct size of blood pressure cuff. If the adult has a very small arm, a pediatric cuff may be necessary. If the resident has a large arm, an extra large size cuff may be necessary. A cuff that is too small for the resident will result in a high reading. A cuff that is too large will result in a low reading.

- Before starting make sure the gauge is properly calibrated. This means that when there is no air in the cuff, the pin should be within the rectangle at the bottom of the gauge. If a gauge is not properly calibrated, it will give an inaccurate reading. Return the cuff to the nurse if it is not calibrated.

- Do not take the blood pressure on an arm that is paralyzed, injured, or the arm on a mastectomy side or an arm with an I.V.

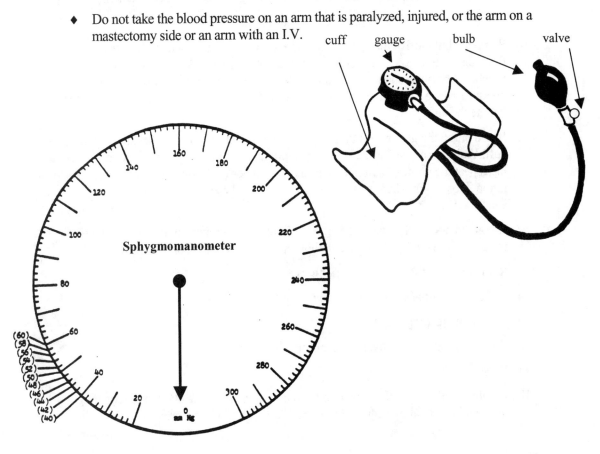

Measuring Blood Pressure

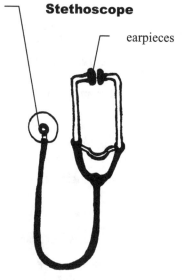

Diaphragm of stethoscope

Stethoscope

earpieces

Procedure:

1. Gather your equipment : alcohol wipes, pen and paper, stethoscope, sphygmomanometer.

2. Clean the **diaphragm of the stethoscope** and earpieces with alcohol wipes.

3. Have the resident sit in a comfortable position with the arm extended and resting with palm up. There should be no clothing on the arm up to the shoulder or rolled up above the BP cuff, and the arm should be above heart level. Place the blood pressure cuff snugly on the resident's upper arm.

4. Position the gauge so you can clearly see it.

5. Turn the valve on the bulb of the sphygmomanometer to the left (counterclockwise) and make sure there is no air in the cuff. If there is, squeeze the air out of the cuff.

6. Turn the valve to the right, clockwise.

7. Feel for the **brachial artery** (1-1 ½ inches above the elbow toward the inside of the elbow) with your fingers. Wrap the cuff snugly above the brachial artery.

8. Put the **diaphragm of the stethoscope** over the brachial artery and hold it in place with your hand. The diaphragm should not be touching the blood pressure cuff.

9. Put the earpieces of the stethoscope in your ears.

10. Pump the bulb to 160mm hg. Open the valve by turning it counter clockwise slowly. The first pulse sound you will hear is the systolic blood pressure. Make a mental note of this number. The pulse sound will continue. When the pulse sound stops, this is the diastolic pressure. Make a mental note of this number. When the sound disappears, completely deflate the cuff.

11. If you pump the gauge to 160mm hg and hear the pulse sound immediately, deflate the cuff. Wait one minute, inflating it to 190mm hg. If your hear the pulse sound at 190mm hg, repeat the process, pumping it 30 mm hg higher to 210mm hg. The objective is to pump it to a point where you do not hear any sound so you are able to determine when the sound starts.

12. If you did not get the reading, wait one minute before repeating the procedure. Check to make sure the diaphragm of the stethoscope is indeed on the brachial artery.

13. Remove the stethoscope from your ears.

14. Deflate the cuff and remove it off the arm.

15. Record the reading.

16. If you are uncertain of the results, check with the charge nurse.

17. Wash your hands.

18. An abnormal BP should be reported verbally to the nurse in addition to recording the information. BP above 140/90 or below 100/60 should be reported.

Chapter 12

Nutrition

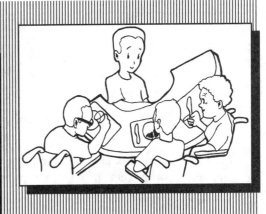

Learning Objectives

1. Explain why good nutrition is important.

2. Describe what your plate should look like at mealtime according to the US Department of Agriculture guidelines for good nutrition.

3. Describe what the following therapeutic diets are: sodium restriction, diabetic, mechanical soft, clear fluids, full fluids, bland, and low residue diet.

4. Explain what aspiration is and what can be done to prevent it.

5. Demonstrate how to feed a resident effectively and safely.

6. List at least 3 things to remember when feeding the dysphagia resident.

7. Explain what the Progressive Self Feeding Program is.

8. List at least 3 adaptive self feeding devices.

9. Record information on flow sheet pertaining to eating.

10. Describe a meal time environment that is conducive to the confused and easily distracted resident.

11. List at least 3 precautions you need to be aware of when taking care of residents with IV, NG, and G tube feeding.

Terms to Know

aspiration
Progressive Self Feeding Program (PSFP)
therapeutic diets
nutrients
proteins
vitamins
minerals
sodium restriction
mechanical soft
clear fluids
full fluids
dysphagia
adaptive self feeding devices
intravenous feeding (IV)
nasogastric feeding (NG)
gastric tube feeding (G tube)

As human beings we have a need for a balanced, nutritious diet. Food provides nourishment to our body through the nutrients it contains. **Nutrients** are chemical substances found in food. Six types of nutrients are: carbohydrates, fats, minerals, proteins, vitamins and water. They are vital to maintain good health Good nutrition is important because it promotes good physical and mental health, promotes healing and resistance to illness and produces energy.

Function and Sources of Nutrients

Proteins are found in meat, milk, eggs, poultry, cheese and fish. They build and renew body tissues and supply energy.

Fats include vegetable oils, butter and can include whole milk and cream, meats, nuts. They provide energy for body activities and energy for body temperature.

Minerals are in milk and milk products, canned salmon and dark green vegetables. They build and renew bones, teeth and regulate activities of muscles, heart, and nerves.

Vitamins include A,B, B1 (Thiamine), B2 (Riboflavin), Niacin B3, B12, C, D. Vitamins perform many services to the body ranging from maintaining healthy condition of skin, hair, nerves, eyes, and digestion, to assisting with general metabolism. There are many food sources that contain different vitamins.

Carbohydrates provide fuel and energy for the body. Carbohydrates include grain products like wheat, pastas, rice, bread and cereals.

Water - A sufficient amount of water and other fluids is essential to maintaining life. Two thirds of our body is water.

Dietary Guidelines

In January 2011, the Department of Agriculture (USDA) issued guidelines for a healthy American diet. The illustration shows what a healthy plate should look like. Half your plate should be fruits and vegetables. Increase the amount of fresh fruits, vegetables, and whole grains in the diet. This is a healthy way to eat and helps a person maintain an ideal weight. Eat foods as close to the way they grew naturally as possible. For example, eat fruits, vegetables, and grains in their natural form instead of processed. Processed foods have more fat and sodium and less fiber and over all nutrition.

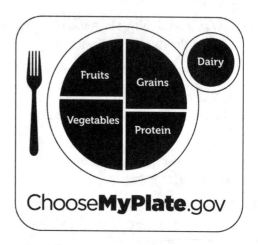

Grains – make at least half your grains whole grains. Whole grains contain the entire grain kernel such as whole-wheat flour, bulgur, oatmeal, and brown rice. Refined grains are milled which gives them a finer texture but also removes much of the fiber and some vitamins. Examples are white flour, white bread, white rice, and pasta. One slice of bread, 1 cup of cereal, or ½ cup of cooked rice or pasta is considered a 1 oz. equivalent from the grains group. For women 3-6 oz. equivalents are recommended per day, for men 4-8 oz. is recommended daily.

Vegetables – they can be cooked, raw, fresh, frozen, dehydrated, canned or 100% juice. There are 5 subgroups of vegetables.

Dark, green vegetable such as broccoli, romaine lettuce, bok choy, collard greens, spinach, etc.

Red and orange vegetables such as squash, carrots, pumpkins, tomatoes, red peppers, etc

Bean and peas such as black beans, white beans, kidney, navy, pinto and garbanzo beans, split peas and lentils

Starchy vegetables such as corn, green peas, green lima beans, potatoes, plantains, etc.

Other vegetables such as artichokes, asparagus, avocado, beets cabbage, cauliflower, eggplants, mushroom, onions, parsnips and zucchini.

One cup of raw or cooked vegetables or vegetable juice or 2 cups of raw leafy greens can be considered as 1 cup from the vegetable group. For women, 2½ cups is recommended daily, for men 3 cups is recommended daily.

Fruit – they can be fresh, canned, frozen, dried or pureed, or 100% fruit juice. Fruits include apples, apricots, bananas, berries, cherries, grapes, mangoes, melons, oranges, peaches, pears, plums, raisins, prunes, pineapple, etc.

One cup of fruit, 1 cup of 100% fruit juice, or ½ cup of dried fruit is considered one cup from the fruit group. For women 1½ cups is recommended daily, for men 2 cups is recommended daily.

Make half your plate fruits and vegetables!

Dairy – includes fluid milk products and foods made from milk. Commonly eaten choices include yogurt, ice cream, hard, soft and processed cheese. Choose fat-free, or low fat milk, yogurt and cheese. One cup of milk, 8 oz. of yogurt, 1½ oz. of hard cheese, or 1/3 cup of shredded cheese or 1 ½ cups of ice cream counts as one cup in the dairy group toward your daily recommended intake. For both men and women, 3 cups are recommended daily.

Protein – foods made from meat, poultry, seafood, beans, peas, eggs, processed soy product, nuts, and seeds are considered part of the protein group. One oz. of meat, poultry or fish, ¼ cup cooked beans, 1 egg, 1 tablespoon of peanut butter or ½ oz. of nuts or seeds are considered os 1 oz. equivalent from the protein group. For women 5-5 ½ oz. is recommended daily, for men 5 ½ -6 oz. is recommended daily.

Limit your intake of trans fats, saturated fats, sugars, salt and alcohol. Saturated fats, trans fats and cholesterol tend to raise "bad" (LDL) cholesterol levels in the blood, which increase risk for heart disease. Coconut oil and palm kernel oil are high in saturated fats. Check the nutritional facts label on food products for trans fats and other contents. Saturated fats are butter, shortening, stick margarine, and animal fats.

Therapeutic Diets

The diet the resident is served in a long term care facility is prescribed by the physician and developed by the dietician. Any resident that has no dietary restrictions is on a regular diet. Some residents need a special diet (therapeutic diet) depending on their medical condition. This **therapeutic diet** is a way of treating a particular medical problem the person may have. For example, maintaining a diabetic diet is very important for the diabetic resident as it can help keep he blood sugar within acceptable limits.

Therapeutic diets include...

Low sodium/salt restriction diet- People who have heart disease, kidney or liver disease, or hypertension may have this diet prescribed. Excess sodium causes the body to retain water which can cause additional problems for these diseases. The physician will prescribe the degree of sodium restriction based on the severity of the condition. The diet can be strict, moderate, or mild restriction. Foods high in sodium are hot dogs, ham, dry cereal, smoked meats, canned foods, etc.. There should be no salt provided on the tray.

Diabetic diet- Personalized for the person with a balance of carbohydrates, fats, proteins and calories. It is important that the person eat at the same time each day to maintain a certain blood suger level.

Mechanical Soft- Foods that are finely chopped assist the resident with chewing and swallowing.

Reducing diet- The calorie count is limited to enable weight loss.

Low residue- Foods low in bulk and fiber

Bland diet- Diet that is non- spicy and mild for easier digestion.

Pureed- Blenderized with little texture.

Low Cholesterol- Diet that limits eggs, butter, whole milk and meats

Low fat- Diet that limits fats such as in meats, oils, eggs, fried foods.

Clear fluids- Fluids that can be "seen through" such as broths, tea, jello. This is meant as a temporary measure such as in preparation for surgery or procedures.

Full fluids- This diet includes any fluids that liquefy at room temperature. This can include broths, ice cream, custards and pudding. This can be a long term diet for people who have difficulty chewing or swallowing.

Mealtime

It is important to make mealtime a pleasant experience for the resident. The dietary staff should work to make the meal visually appealing to the resident. The meal should be served in an environment that is calm, soothing, free of odors and noisy distractions. The resident should be allowed to eat in a non-rushed manner and supervised for safety. While the resident is eating, a care giver should be present who observes for any signs of choking. Every effort should be made to distribute the trays promptly so the food reaches the resident at optimal temperature, that is, hot foods hot, cold food cold. If the resident tells you about strong food preferences or dislikes, please pass this on to the dietary staff.

Proper Position for Eating or Drinking

Incorrect Position for Eating or Drinking

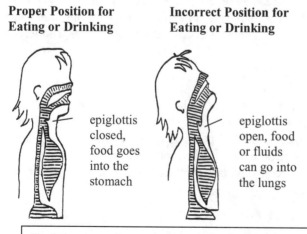

epiglottis closed, food goes into the stomach

epiglottis open, food or fluids can go into the lungs

Residents must be properly positioned. This means sitting in a straight, 90^0 upright position. This is to prevent **aspiration** which means inhaling food or fluids into the lungs. This can lead to deadly aspiration pneumonia. If the resident eats or drinks with their head extended back, this automatically opens up the epiglottis. The epiglottis is the trap door that leads to the lungs. If a person eats or drinks with the epiglottis open, they can aspirate food or fluids into their lungs.

Feed the **stomach**, not the **lungs**. Don't allow the head to tilt back because this throws all the swallowing mechanism out of line.

Adaptive Self-Feeding Devices

These are special utensils and devices that can assist the resident in helping themselves despite their disabilities. The occupational therapist will evaluate the resident and make recommendations for specific devices such as...

Rolling knife that looks like a little pizza cutter. This can enable a resident to cut their food with use of only one hand.

A spork which is a combination spoon and fork (a spoon with 3 points).

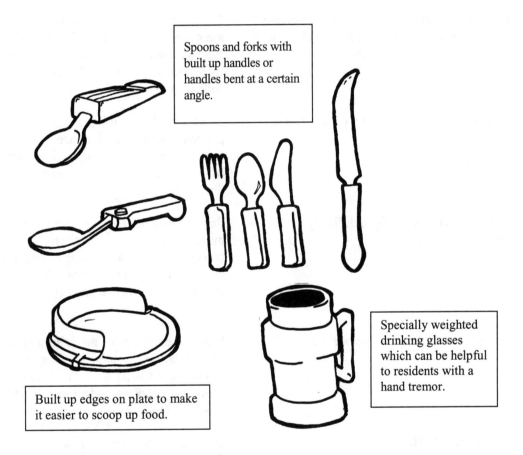

Spoons and forks with built up handles or handles bent at a certain angle.

Specially weighted drinking glasses which can be helpful to residents with a hand tremor.

Built up edges on plate to make it easier to scoop up food.

Progressive Self Feeding Program

This is a special program where a small group of residents under supervision of staff, work toward re-learning to feed themselves. The ultimate goal is eventual self feeding. The resident is supervised and assisted as needed. The environment should be quiet, non-distracting and supportive.

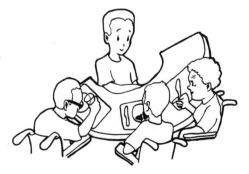

Insuring Adequate Nutrition

Some of your residents may present a challenge as far as nutrition and feeding is concerned.

Some residents may...

Not be able to feed themselves due to paralysis, weakness, dementia or blindness.

What you can do...

You may need to partially assist them in eating. Check with your charge nurse and the flow sheet. Observe the resident and be responsive to their needs. For some, the Progressive Self Feeding Program may be helpful. Adaptive self feeding devices may benefit some residents.

Have difficulty swallowing, thereby presenting a risk for choking and/or aspiration or not being able to take in adequate nutrition.

Position bolt upright while feeding to prevent aspiration. Check with the charge nurse and dietitian. Some foods and types of diet are easier for residents with swallowing difficulties. (See section on dysphagia)

Have missing teeth or dentures or poor fitting dentures.

Check with the charge nurse regarding this problem. He or she can arrange for a dental examination. Dentures may need to be re-adjusted or new dentures may need to be ordered if possible.

Be easily distracted and have difficulty concentrating on eating.

Resident may need to be re-directed at meal time by verbal clues. Talk the resident through the process such as "open", "chew", "swallow". A quiet, not overly noisy or overly stimulating environment can help them focus on the job at hand.

Be agitated, combative and refuse to eat.

Feed the resident in a quiet, calm environment, in a non-hurried manner. They may be over-stimulated in a large, noisy dining room. Be reassuring and non-threatening and allow them to set the pace.

Have a poor appetite.

Observe and ask what their food preferences are. Talk with the charge nurse and dietary staff in an effort to accommodate them. Report to the nurse if the resident has not completed at least 60% of the meal. A meal replacement nourishment will be offered the resident as directed by the nurse. It is important that the resident maintain good nutritional intake.

Procedure: Feeding the Dependent Resident

Wash your hands.

Make sure the resident has clean hands, face, and brushed teeth. If resident wears dentures, make sure that they are in the mouth. The resident must be awake, alert and responsive. Do not force the resident to eat.

Position the resident at a 90^0 upright position. Make sure they have a napkin and clothing protector.

Check the resident diet card against resident ID to make sure the correct meal is being served.

Season the meal as the resident requests and as the diet allows.

Sit down at the eye level of the resident and tell them what you are about to do.

Keep all requests to the resident simple, ("open your mouth, chew, swallow").

If the resident cannot see, tell them which food item you are feeding them. Some residents may be partially or totally blind, have poor peripheral vision (vision out of corner of eyes) or have visual field cuts (sections of vision missing). In describing what is on their plate to them you can use a clock as a description of what is on the plate. An example is "your meatloaf is at 2 o'clock, your carrots are at 5 o'clock, your potatoes are at 7 o'clock, your bread at 10 o'clock. They can visualize where the food items are on the plate and can feed themselves better.

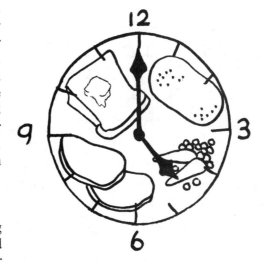

Tuck a napkin under their chin.

Fill the spoon half full and enter the mouth using the tip of the spoon. Alternate types of food offered allowing for resident's preferences. Offer food in bite size pieces. Make sure the resident's mouth is empty before next bite or sip of fluid.

Offer fluids periodically to help wash down the food. Make sure the fluids are not too hot.

Talk with the resident throughout the meal.

Allow the resident plenty of time for chewing and swallowing. Watch the Adam's apple rising and falling as indication of swallowing. Let the resident set the pace for feeding.

Help the resident wipe his mouth and hands with the napkin as needed. Make sure the resident is clean after completing the meal. Remove and discard the clothing protector in the proper container.

Allow the resident to sit upright for at least 30 minutes after eating to prevent aspiration.

Remove the food tray.

Document what the resident has eaten and if indicated what fluids the resident consumed. Notify the nurse if the resident has not finished at least 60% of the meal. If the resident is to have intake and output documented, do so.

Leave the resident in a comfortable and safe position with the call light within easy reach.

Wash your hands.

Resident's Name _____ **Room #** _____ **Month** _____ **Year** _____

		1	2	3	4	5	6	7	8	9	10	11	12	13	14	15	16	17	18	19	20	21	22	23	24	25	26	27	28	29	30	31
Initial for Meal Monitor	Breakfast																															
	Lunch																															
	Dinner																															
Chart % of Meal Eaten	Breakfast																															
	Lunch																															
	Dinner																															
If Less than 75% of Meal Eaten, Offer 200cc of Nourishment Chart cc's Taken	Breakfast																															
	Lunch																															
	Dinner																															
If Less Than 100 cc's of Nourishment Taken, Notify Licensed Nurse and Initial	Breakfast																															
	Lunch																															
	Dinner																															
		1	2	3	4	5	6	7	8	9	10	11	12	13	14	15	16	17	18	19	20	21	22	23	24	25	26	27	28	29	30	31

Dysphagia Management

Dysphagia means difficulty swallowing. People who may have dysphagia are stroke and head injury patients, or have Parkinson's disease or multiple sclerosis. Residents with dysphagia are at added risk of aspiration, which can be deadly. Feed residents carefully to avoid aspiration. Indicators of a swallowing disorder may include coughing or choking before, during or after the swallow, food remaining in the mouth after swallowing, complaints of food caught in the throat, excessive mouth movement during chewing and swallowing and difficulty starting a swallow.

Foods that may be difficult to swallow...

Pureed or osterized foods
Sticky foods such as mashed potatoes
Thin liquids such as water

Dry foods such as toast and crackers
Foods that are room temperature or lukewarm

The speech pathologist is the rehabilitation specialist who can be an excellent resource person regarding swallowing difficulties. They may be involved in directing care regarding this problem and may have specific directions on the flow sheet for you or posted at the bedside.

The use of food thickeners may be recommended for dysphagia residents. At mealtime you will need to add the thickener according to directions, perhaps adding it to juice to make it thicker. This makes it easier and safer to swallow. Hot foods (but not so hot as to burn) and cold foods like milkshakes are easier to swallow.

Feeding the resident with dysphagia...

1. Resident should be sitting straight upright.

2. Do not rush resident, if possible allow resident to "pace" eating.

3. If residents fatigue rapidly, they may need smaller, more frequent meals.

4. Provide verbal "cues" to remind resident to "open", "chew", and "swallow".

5. Avoid distractions, resident must concentrate to swallow.

6. Watch Adams apple rising and falling as indication of swallowing.

7. Capitalize on sensory awareness in terms of taste, texture and temperature.

8. Residents may "pocket" food in their cheeks. Check the mouth carefully including the cheeks, under the tongue and on the roof of the mouth when they are done eating.

9. Do not put the resident in a reclining position for at least 30 minutes after eating, to avoid aspiration.

Alternative Feeding Methods

There are residents who cannot eat solid foods and must be fed in another way. Although the nursing assistant does not administer these feedings, you need to have an understanding of them.

Intravenous (I.V.) feedings - a bag of sterile liquid, medications, or nutrient solution flows through a plastic cannula and needle into the vein. The amount of fluids and the type are prescribed by the physician and administered by the RN.

Things to remember when taking care of a resident with an I.V.

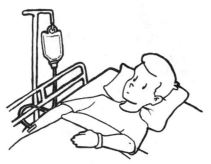

1. When moving or transferring the resident, make sure there is no pulling on the tubing. A portable I.V. stand is used when the resident ambulates.

2. Do not in any way change or stop the infusion of the fluid. Report if the rate changes or stops.

3. Make sure the tubing is not pinched or kinked and that the resident is not lying on it or pulling it.

4. Report if the pump alarm sounds.

5. Observe for and report if you see redness, swelling, leaking or bleeding at the insertion site, or complaints of pain at the site of insertion.

6. Report to the nurse if the resident has elevated temperature, chest pain, shortness of breath, loss of consciousness, irregular pulse, hypotension, decrease in urinary output, nausea, or confusion.

7. Do not take the resident's blood pressure on the arm that has an I.V.

8. Notify the nurse if the IV bag is empty or almost empty.

Hyperalimentation or total parenteral nutrition (TPN) - an intravenous catheter is inserted into the subclavian vein in the chest and through the veins of the superior vena cava of the heart. This allows the feedings to bypass the digestive system, allowing it to heal and/or not be stressed. There are many serious risks associated with hyperalimentation. Watch for and report fever, chills, chest pain, tachycardia, shortness of breath, and confusion.

Nasogastric (NG) tube feeding - is used for the resident who cannot swallow or has specific medical problems. The NG tube goes from the nose, through the esophagus to the stomach. The type of feeding and amount is prescribed by the physician and administered by the licensed nurse. Residents require frequent oral care and careful cleaning at the nose where the tube is placed.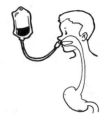

Gastrostomy tube (G) tube feeding - is surgically inserted through the abdominal wall into the stomach. Frequently the feeding is done by pump over a prolonged period of time. The head of the bed must be kept elevated at least 45° while the feeding is running and up to 60 minutes after completion. If the feedings are continuous, the head of the bed must be elevated at all times. Observe the skin for signs of irritation where the tube enters the body.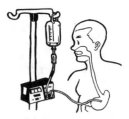

People who have feeding tubes are usually NPO. They may have a dry mouth, dry lips, coated tongue, and generally a bad taste in their mouth. Good oral hygiene and a lubricant to the lips is important. If they have a tube that goes in through the nose you should clean around the nostrils every 4 hours. Observe and report any irration around the nostrils.

With tube feedings but especially with TPN, it is very important not to kink or dislodge the tubing. Move the resident carefully and make sure there is no pulling or pressure against the tubing. When taking care of a resident with a subclavian line, such as the TPN resident, there are some very special precautions you will need to take that the charge nurse will inform you of.

Some residents may experience tube feeding complications. Watch for the following signs and report them to your charge nurse.

Nausea, vomiting, diarrhea

Distended stomach

Constipation and/or cramping

Pain, redness, swelling, heat, crusty or oozing fluids at the site where the feeding tube enters the body.

Cough

Sore throat

Resident has pulled out the tube.

Chapter 12 - Quiz Yourself

Choose the one correct answer.

1. A resident with dysphagia is at added risk of...

    a. stroke
    b. paralysis
    c. swallowing
    d. aspiration

2. Which foods are more difficult to swallow for a resident with dysphagia?

    a. meat loaf, creamed corn
    b. water, mashed potatoes, toast
    c. apricot nectar, milk shake

3. After a dysphagia resident has eaten, do not put them in a flat reclining position for at least...

    a. 30 minutes
    b. 5 minutes
    c. 10 minutes
    d. 2 hours

4. Which of the following statements is false?

    a. Dietary recommendations vary according to our weight, age, and gender.
    b. Trans fats and saturated fats can increase the risk of heart disease.
    c. It is better to eat foods in their natural form instead of processed foods.
    d. Refined grains such as white flour and white rice are better for you than whole grains such as brown rice, cracked wheat, and whole wheat flour.

5. Foods that are high in sodium are...

    a. hot dogs
    b. ham
    c. canned foods
    d. all of the above

True or False

6. _____ You should report to the nurse if the resident has not completed at least 60% of their meal.

7. _____ Sources of protein are milk, meat, cheese, chicken, and eggs.

8. _____ A rehabilitation specialist who is very helpful in dealing with residents who have dysphagia is the speech pathologist.

9. _____ The rehabilitation specialist who is helpful in obtaining adaptive eating devices is the occupational therapist.

10. _____ If a resident has an I.V., it is okay to take the blood pressure on the arm where the I.V. is.

11. _____ It is okay to offer a resident with a nasogastric tube, fluids or food by mouth.

12. _____ The nursing assistant administers NG or G tube feedings.

13. _____ The resident with a feeding tube should not lie flat in bed.

Answer and Explain

14. Mrs. Clark had a stroke with dysphagia. Explain 3 things you need to remember when feeding her at mealtime.

_____

_____

_____

15. Mrs. Clark, who has use of only one hand, is improving and is starting to feed herself. She may benefit from adaptive eating devices. Describe at least 2 adaptive devices that may help her.

_____

_____

16. Describe an ideal eating environment that would benefit the dementia resident.

_____

_____

17. Miss K. has an intravenous feeding. Name 3 abnormalities you should observe for at the insertion site (where the needle goes into the body).

_____

_____

_____

Chapter 13

Fluids - Intake and Output

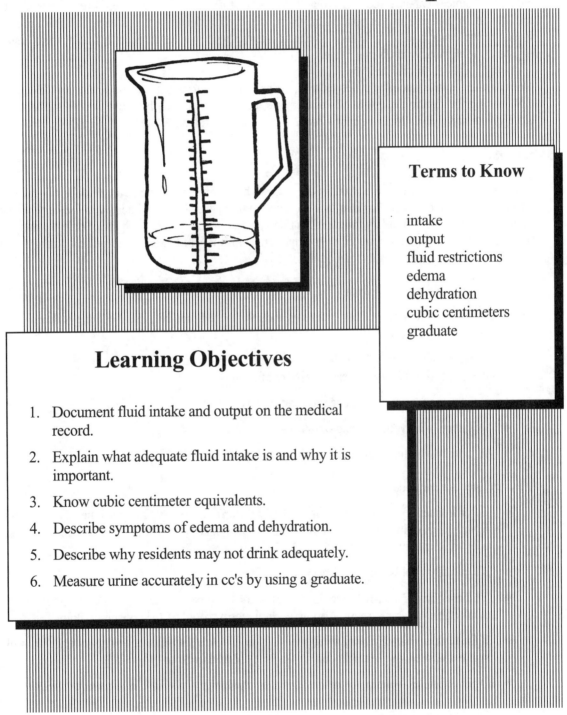

Terms to Know

intake
output
fluid restrictions
edema
dehydration
cubic centimeters
graduate

Learning Objectives

1. Document fluid intake and output on the medical record.

2. Explain what adequate fluid intake is and why it is important.

3. Know cubic centimeter equivalents.

4. Describe symptoms of edema and dehydration.

5. Describe why residents may not drink adequately.

6. Measure urine accurately in cc's by using a graduate.

Need for Fluids

Two thirds (2/3) of our bodies are made up of water. Water helps regulate body temperature, fluid balance, chemical balance and is the major component of blood. Water, therefore, is essential to life. An important part of your job is to insure that the resident maintains adequate fluid intake. Fluids mean water and other liquids. If the resident does not take in enough fluids, the nursing assistant should notify the charge nurse.

Normal fluid intake should be between 2,500 and 3,000 cubic centimeters (cc's) per day, with 2,500 being the minimum. 1,000 cc's equals one quart, therefore, daily intake should be between 2.5 and 3 quarts daily. Fluids taken in (intake) and fluids excreted (output) should roughly be equal.

Dehydration

Dehydration means inadequate fluid in the body. This can occur if the resident does not take in adequate amounts of fluids, has diarrhea and/or vomiting. The flu can be deadly in the very young or elderly because of vomiting and diarrhea that can lead to dehydration. Signs of dehydration are weakness, dry mouth, concentrated dark urine, cracked lips, confusion, rapid pulse, lethargy, and low blood pressure. Dehydration can be deadly!

Residents who are at risk of dehydration

- ♦ Residents who have kidney problems and lose more fluids because the kidneys do not concentrate urine as well.

- ♦ Residents who do not have the ability to pour themselves fluids or drink independently due to paralysis, muscle weakness, or confusion.

- ♦ Residents who are on diuretic medications (water pills).

- ♦ Residents with vomiting and/or diarrhea.

- ♦ Residents who have difficulty swallowing liquids.

Ways to Encourage Fluids

- ♦ Offer frequent opportunities to drink fluids. Offer fluids every time you enter the resident's room. Many elderly do not feel thirst the way younger people do, therefore, will not drink adequate amounts on their own.

- ♦ Keep fresh, cool water within easy reach of the resident.

- ♦ You may hear the term "force fluids". This does not mean to actually force a person to drink against his or her will. A more accurate term would be to "encourage fluids".

- ♦ If the resident has difficulty swallowing, offer "thicker" liquids such as apricot nectar, milk shakes, slushes, or use thickeners in fluids if ordered to do so.

- ♦ Offer popsicles, gelatin, ice cream, and fruit slushes if allowed. These count as fluids.

Edema

Edema is fluid retention in the tissues, particularly of the hands and feet. It occurs when fluid output is less than fluid intake. Edema may occur due to congestive heart failure, kidney diseases, or other diseases.

If a person has edema it is a good idea to keep legs elevated part of the day. Ambulation stimulates circulation which helps relieve edema. Additionally, a physician may prescribe compression stockings.

Some residents may have physician's orders to restrict the amount of fluids they can consume, due to heart or kidney disease. You will be informed as to how much fluids the resident is allowed on your shift. Usually the day shift is allowed the largest quantity, evening shift less, and the night shift the least. All intake will need to be documented on the intake and output sheet.

Measuring Intake and Output

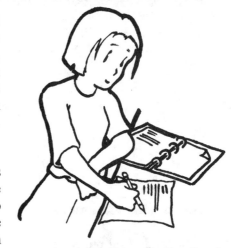

There are some residents who will require careful monitoring of intake and output (I & O). **Intake** means fluids that are taken in, either by mouth, through nasogastric (NG) tube feedings, or through intravenous (I.V.) feedings. Fluids are liquids such as water, juices and any substances that liquefy at room temperature such as ice cream, custard and puddings. **Output** means urine, vomitus, and any drainage.

When you are told to **record intake and output**, this means to keep an accurate record of all fluids that are taken in and all fluids eliminated. You will need to record intake on the I & O sheet. Either at the top of the I & O sheet or on a separate sheet, you will be given cubic centimeter equivalents of such things as juice glass, soup bowl, etc. Immediately after the resident completes drinking or eating, write down the amount taken in. Do not trust your memory for later documentation. If the resident is capable, have them write down everything they drink. The charge nurse will maintain records of intake via tube feedings, or I.V. solutions.

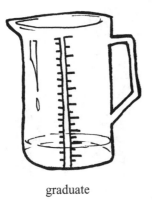

graduate

Measure output immediately after it occurs. A resident may void into a **specimen pan** or a urinal which has measurements written on the side in cc's and ounces. Urine can also be poured into a **graduate**, which is a measuring device. Read the measurement at eye level and record it on the I & O sheet. Your nursing supervisor will help you estimate any output by drainage or emesis.

Intake and output totals will be added up at the end of each shift and also at the end of the 24 hour period.

I & O results will be evaluated by the charge nurse for the valuable information they provide.

There will be times when the charge nurse will determine that a record of what the resident takes in (intake) and puts out (output) will need to be observed and documented. This may include...

- ◆ on admission of the resident for a few days
- ◆ when the resident is on certain medications
- ◆ if there is concern about dehydration or edema

How to Calculate cc's

A cubic centimeter is a unit of measure and is equal to 1 milliliter.

1 oz. = 30 cc or 30 ml.

If you are calculating intake, know the amount of ounces and multiply by 30 cc's.

For example...   8 oz. = 240 cc (8 x 30 cc's)   10 oz. = 300 cc (10 x 30 cc's)

1 milliliter (ml.)	=	1 cubic centimeter (cc)
1 teaspoon	=	5 cc
1 oz.	=	30 cc or 30 ml.
1 pint	=	500 cc
1 quart	=	1000 cc
1 gallon	=	4000 cc

Calculating Measurements

Your facility will provide you measurements in cc's of the cups, glasses and bowls used. The following are sample measurements but could vary from facility to facility.

coffee cup   120 cc

milk carton   240 cc

small juice glass   120 cc

paper cup   150 cc

soup bowl   160 cc

ice cream container   120 cc

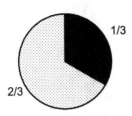

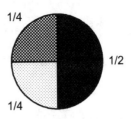

When calculating intake you need to understand fractions.

How many cc's are in the following?

8 oz.   =_____cc.   1/2 of milk carton   =_____cc

3 oz.   =_____cc.   1/4 of juice glass   =_____cc

5 oz.   =_____cc.   1/3 of coffee cup   =_____cc

2 qts.   =_____cc.

Procedure: Measuring Output

Prepare equipment and supplies: disposable gloves, bedpan, graduate container.

1.   Wash hands and put on gloves before handling bedpan.

2.   Pour the contents of the bedpan into the measuring (graduate) container.

3.   While keeping the container level, measure the amount of urine.

4.   Empty contents of measuring container into the toilet.

5.   Return bedpan and measuring container to proper storage.

6.   Remove and dispose of gloves.

7.   Wash your hands.

8.   Record output in cc's.

INTAKE AND OUTPUT RECORD

Resident_____

Room Number_____ Date_____

INTAKE	OUTPUT
10:30 - 6:30 AM	10:30 - 6:30 AM
6:30 - 2:30 PM	6:30 - 2:30 PM
2:30 - 10:30 PM	2:30 - 10:30 PM

24 hour totals   INTAKE   24 hours totals   OUTPUT

URINE IN BRIEFS

small amount	75 cc
moderate amount	200 cc
very large amount	300 cc

Chapter 13 - Quiz Yourself

True or False

1. _____ To force fluids means to force a resident to drink whether they want to or not.

2. _____ A graduate is used to measure fluids in cc's.

3. _____ Fluids are important because they help regulate body temperature.

4. _____ Ice cream, jello, sherbet and pudding are considered fluids.

5. _____ It is acceptable to rely on your memory and write down the intake and output numbers at the end of your shift rather than writing it down immediately after a meal.

6. _____ Urinary drainage bags should be emptied at the end of each shift.

Give equivalent measurements.

7. 18 oz.   = _____cc.

8. 12 oz.   = _____cc.

9. 2 cc   = _____ml.

10. List 3 symptoms of dehydration.

_____

_____

_____

11. Give 3 reasons why residents may not drink adequately.

_____

_____

_____

Choose the one correct answer.

12. Mrs. Jones has fluid retention in her hands and legs, with a 3 lb. weight gain this last week. This is called...

    a. fat
    b. edema
    c. dehydration
    d. hemiporesis

13. 2500 cc is equal to...

    a. 1 quart
    b. 1 1/2 quarts
    c. 2 1/2 quarts
    d. 1 gallon

Chapter 14

The Gastro-Intestinal and Urinary Systems

Learning Objectives

1. Explain the aging changes that occur regarding the urinary and digestive systems

2. Explain the main functions of small and large intestines, and stomach.

3. Explain the main function of the urethra, bladder, and ureters.

4. Describe special precautions required when doing peri-care.

5. Identify three observations the caregiver would make and report to the nurse regarding urine and stool.

6. Describe what constipation and impaction are.

7. Identify at least 3 signs and symptoms of a urinary tract infection.

8. Demonstrate how to assist resident onto commode and bedpan.

9. Describe the different types of incontinence.

10. Demonstrate peri-care for the resident with an indwelling Foley catheter.

11. Explain what a bowel and bladder re-training program is.

Terms to Know

commode
small intestine
large intestine
meatus
(UTI) urinary tract infection
stomach
kidneys
ureters
bladder
urethra
catheter
catheterization
incontinent
void
anus
Foley catheter
condom catheter
fracture pan
bedpan
urinate
elimination
feces
defecation
stool
diarrhea
impaction
constipation
colostomy
ileostomy
stomach

These Are Four Steps You Must Take Before Starting Any Procedure

1. Wash your hands and use standard precautions including wearing gloves when appropriate.

2. Identify yourself to the resident and call them by name. Check their wrist band to establish identity.

3. Explain the procedure to the resident speaking clearly, slowly and directly while maintaining face to face contact whenever possible.

4. Provide privacy by closing doors, pulling privacy curtains, closing drapes or blinds.

End all procedures by doing the following...

1. Discard gloves if used.

2. Wash your hands.

3. Leave call signal within reach of resident.

4. Make sure that the resident is left in a safe and comfortable position.

The Urinary System

The functions of the urinary system are...

♦ remove waste from the bloodstream

♦ produce urine

♦ maintain homeostasis (a balance of systems in the body)

The urinary system is comprised of...

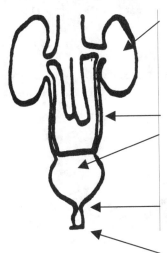

Kidneys - two bean shaped organs that lie just below the diaphragm and posterior (back) abdominal wall on either side of the spine. The kidneys contain over a million microscopic filtering units called nephrons. Waste products are separated from the blood and along with excess fluids create urine.

Ureters - two long tubes which connect the kidneys with the bladder.

Bladder - a hollow muscular organ for storage of urine. Stretch receptor nerve cells become stimulated when the bladder is full and sends a message to the brain which results in urination.

Urethra - a tube through which urine runs from the bladder to the outside of the body. Infections from the outside of the body can enter through here and infect the bladder or even the kidneys.

Meatus - exterior opening into urinary tract.

Adequate fluid intake is important to maintain normal kidney functioning. The kidneys determine the water and chemical composition of the blood which determines the content of the tissue fluid that surrounds cells.

Urinary Changes That Occur With Aging

There is less blood flow to the kidneys so that the kidney tissue does not receive enough nutrients and oxygen. This causes further destruction of kidney tissue. Also, since waste products are brought to the kidney in the blood, this process does not work as well.

The bladder becomes less elastic, which means it cannot stretch as much as it used to. The result is that the bladder cannot hold as much urine as it used to, and the person needs to go to the bathroom more frequently.

The muscles which close off the urethra and thereby prevent unwanted urination, do not function as well as in the past. Older people often complain of "dribbling". Additionally they have to urinate more often than they previously did. This can be annoying, especially if they have to get up several times during the night. Accidents are more likely to happen when the resident gets up in the night with sudden position change which may result in dizziness.

The bladder may not empty completely. This is especially true if the resident is not sitting bolt upright. This can lead to urinary tract infection.

Urinary Elimination

Elimination is something we all need to do every few hours. It is also a very private act. Many of the residents rely on the care givers to assist them with their elimination needs. It is important to protect the resident's privacy by pulling curtains, closing doors, pulling shades etc., while still insuring that they are safe. You may need to stand outside the bathroom door maintaining voice contact to insure that the resident is fine or stand on the other side of the privacy curtain. Some resident however may be weak and disabled and will need your constant presence there during elimination.

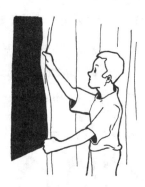

Bedpans

Some residents may not be able to get out of bed to **urinate or void** (to pass urine). Women use **bedpans** for urination and bowel movements. Men use bedpans for bowel movements and **urinals** for urination.

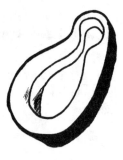

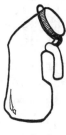

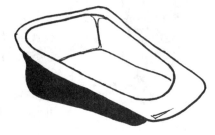

urinal

fracture pan

bedpan

Fracture pans are used for residents who cannot move or bend much or for those that have casts or are in traction. They are smaller with thinner rims. The smaller end goes under the buttocks.

When handling bedpans it is important to use standard precautions. Keep the bedpan covered when taking it to the toilet, dirty utility room or out in the hall. Disinfect the bedpan and return it to the bedside stand with a clean cover.

Procedure: Giving Resident the Bedpan

Assemble the following equipment: bedpan, cover for bedpan, disposable gloves, toilet tissue, hand wipes, protective pad.

1. Provide for privacy.

2. Position the resident in a supine position with the head of the bed lowered. Place a protective pad under resident's buttocks to protect bed linens.

3. Put on clean gloves before handling bedpan.

4. If the resident is able, ask them to raise buttocks and slide the bedpan underneath.

5. If the resident cannot raise buttocks, turn the resident on side away from you. Place the bedpan against the buttocks and while holding the bedpan securely, turn the resident onto it.

6. With the standard bedpan, position the bedpan so the wider end of the pan is aligned with the resident's buttocks. With the fracture pan, position the bedpan with the resident sitting on the lower end of the bedpan.

7. Remove and dispose of gloves into waste container and wash hands.

8. Cover the resident with linen for warmth and privacy. Avoid any unnecessary exposure of the resident throughout the procedure.

9. Raise the head of the bed.

10. Leave the toilet tissue and signaling device within reach of the resident. Ask the resident to use the signaling device when they are finished.

11. Leave hand wipes within reach and instruct resident to clean hands when finished.

12. When resident has used the bedpan put on clean gloves.

13. Lower the head of the bed before removing the bedpan. Ask the resident to raise buttocks. If the resident cannot raise buttocks, turn on side away from you and remove the bedpan.

14. Provide perineal care if the resident cannot clean own genital area.

15. Remove the bedpan, empty contents into the toilet. Rinse the bedpan, pouring rinse water into the toilet and return the bedpan to proper storage.

16. Remove and discard the gloves without contaminating yourself. Wash your hands.

17. Return the resident to a comfortable and safe position.

18. Leave the signaling device within reach of the resident. Leave the bed in the lowered position.

19. Pull back the privacy curtain.

20. Wash your hands.

21. Report pertinent observations to your charge nurse.

Commode Chair

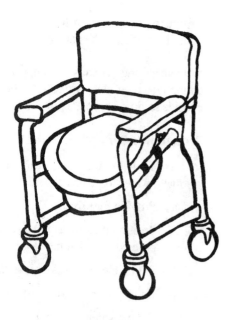

Some residents may not be able to get to the bathroom easily and may need to use the commode at the bedside. A **commode** is a portable bedside toilet. As usual, provide for privacy while the resident is being transferred to the commode and while using it. Use good transfer techniques in helping the resident transfer from the bed to the commode and vice versa. When the resident has used the commode chair, remove and empty the receptacle, being sure to keep it covered while in route to the bathroom. Use disposable gloves when handling the receptacle. Observe the urine and stool and report to the nurse if there is anything unusual. Save a sample for the nurse to see if that is the case. Clean and disinfect the receptacle according to facility policy and store appropriately.

Urinary Catheters

Catheters are only used as prescribed by the physician for very specific needs. Catheters (except the condom catheter) provide a direct opening into the bladder, thus allowing the possibility of very serious infections. They, therefore, are prescribed only when absolutely necessary and never for the convenience of the staff. They may be necessary in the following situations...

♦ After surgery when the person cannot empty their bladder on their own.

♦ Due to neurological conditions where the person cannot feel the need to empty the bladder nor be able to empty the bladder.

♦ Residents who retain urine until the bladder is stretched beyond comfortable capacity.

There are two types of catheters, external and internal. The external catheter is known as a **condom catheter** and fits over a man's penis and drains into a drainage bag. There are three types of internal catheters.

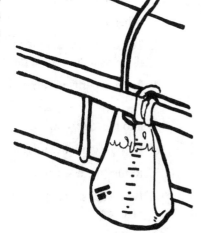

♦ Indwelling urethral catheter (**Foley catheter**) inserted by the RN or LPN using sterile technique through the urethra into the bladder to drain off urine into the drainage bag.

♦ Indwelling suprapubic catheter placed by RN or LPN directly into the bladder through an opening into the abdomen above the pubic bone. The catheter attached to the tubing drains the urine into the drainage bag.

♦ Straight catheter inserted by the RN or LPN using sterile technique through the urethra into the bladder to drain urine. It is used to obtain a sterile urine specimen and then removed.

Nursing Assistant Responsibilities Regarding Catheter Care

Apply gloves before handling the catheter.

Be certain all connections are tight to prevent leakage from the catheter and prevent germs from entering the drainage system. Do not disconnect the tubing. Attach the tubing to the bed with a plastic clip.

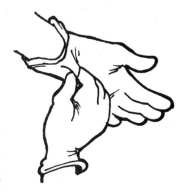

Make sure the tubing is free of kinks and that the urine is flowing freely.

Make sure the drainage bag is below the level of the catheter and bladder and is attached to the frame of the bed not the side rail. It should never touch the floor.

Report to the nurse if there is any leaking around the catheter. This can be a sign of obstruction, bladder spasms or UTI (urinary tract infection).

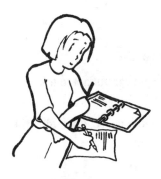

Report any complaints of pain or discomfort.

Catheters should be taped to the inside of the leg to prevent pulling on the bladder.

Careful intake and output records must be maintained. A fluid intake of at least 2500 cc. per day is desirable.

Notify the charge nurse immediately if there is decreased urinary output. Most residents will have between 50-80 cc. per hour output.

Notify the nurse immediately if the urine appears to be particularly dark, foul-smelling or have sediment in the catheter tubing.

Move and transfer the resident carefully so as not to dislodge the catheter by pulling on the tubing.

Condom Catheter Care

A condom catheter may be used for a male resident. Prior to application of the condom catheter, perineal care must be done. Roll the catheter onto the penis moving from the end of the penis toward the body leaving a one inch space between the penis and the end of the catheter. The catheter needs to be taped to the inside thigh to prevent pulling on the catheter. The condom catheter must be removed at least once daily for perineal care. Observe and report any redness, swelling or discomfort to the charge nurse.

Procedure: Emptying the Urinary Drainage Bag

1. Assemble equipment as necessary: disposable gloves, graduate (measuring cup that shows cc's).

2. Put on gloves.

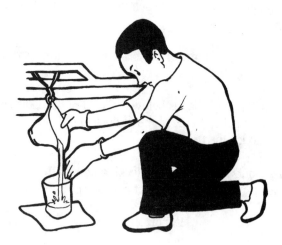

3. Place the graduate so the urine can be collected when drain is opened.

4. Open the drainage spout at the bottom of the drainage bag, being careful not to touch the tip of the spout itself.

5. Without letting the spout touch the sides of the graduate or anything else, drain the urine into the graduate.

6. Close the spout and replace it in the holder on the bag.

7. Measure the urinary output. Observe for color and character of the urine.

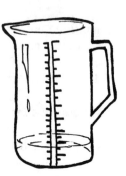

8. Discard the urine.

9. Disinfect the graduate and return it to its proper place.

10. Remove and dispose of your gloves and wash your hands.

11. Record the time and output in cc's on the I&O record.

12. Report any pertinent observations to your charge nurse

Procedure: Catheter Care

1. Assemble equipment necessary: disposable gloves, bed protector, wash basin, warm water, soap or peri-care solution, towels, wash cloth.

2. Cover the resident with a bath blanket and fan-fold top linen at the foot of the bed.

3. Test the water in the basin to determine that it is safe and comfortable for the resident.

4. Wash your hands and put on your disposable gloves.

5. Put disposable bed protector under the buttocks.

6. Expose the area surrounding catheter only. Provide for privacy throughout the procedure.

7. Apply soap to the washcloth.

8. Hold the catheter near the meatus (exterior opening to the urinary tract) to avoid tugging.

9. Clean at least 4 inches of the catheter closest to the meatus moving in only one direction (away from the meatus) using a clean area of cloth for each stroke. Avoid tugging on the catheter.

10. Rinse at least 4 inches of the catheter closest to the meatus moving in only one direction (away from the meatus) using a clean area of the cloth for each stroke. Avoid tugging on the catheter.

11. Dry at least 4 inches of the catheter closest to the meatus, moving away from the meatus.

12. Secure the catheter by taping it to the inner thigh.

13. Empty, rinse, and wipe the basin and return it to the proper storage.

14. Remove the bed protector. Dispose of linen in proper containers. Avoid touching soiled linen to your clothing.

15. Remove and discard gloves. Wash your hands.

16. Make sure the resident is comfortable. Leave the bed in lowest position.

17. Leave the signaling device within reach of the resident.

Urinary Tract Infection (UTI)

A urinary tract infection can be a potentially serious infection. It can cause serious complications, especially in the elderly. It can develop into bacteremia (infection in the blood stream) which in some people can prove deadly. It therefore is important to be observant for possible signs and symptoms of a UTI and for this information to be quickly reported to the charge nurse. A sample of urine can be sent to the laboratory for analysis (urinalysis) and the specific infection and treatment identified (culture and sensitivity). It is important for the resident to be quickly started on antibiotics to treat the infection.

The following may be signs and symptoms of a urinary tract infection (UTI)

Dark, cloudy urine

Strong, foul smelling urine

Sediment, or particles in urine

Complaints of burning on urination

Complaints of pain on urination

Trouble starting urinary stream

Incontinence

Change in behavior such as disorientation and restlessness

Sensation of needing to urinate frequently

Many elderly may not feel physical discomfort

Things you can do to decrease infection

Encourage adequate fluids, at least 2,500 cc., unless contraindicated (not advised) by the physician.

Maintain clean perineal condition. When doing peri-care, wipe carefully from front to back, being careful not to introduce any fecal matter from around the rectum to the urethra.

Juices that are acidic such as cranberry juice can make the urine Ph acidic which is a hostile environment for bacteria growth.

Incontinence

Urinary incontinence is the inability to control the passage of urine from the bladder. It unfortunately is a problem that affects many of our residents. It causes discomfort, odors, potential skin irritation, pressure areas and is embarrassing to the resident. The resident who is incontinent needs to be changed promptly and receive careful peri care to wash away all traces of urine. Many people cannot control when or where they urinate. This is not a normal part of aging but many residents have this problem.

Different types of incontinence

Some residents may not be aware that their bladders are full, such as residents who have dementia, spinal cord injuries or central nervous system damage. Their bladders empty automatically.

Some residents may have **stress incontinence**. The person may dribble or release urine when they sneeze, cough or laugh, exercise or move in a certain way. Women often have stress incontinence.

Some residents may have **urge incontinence.** The person may have little warning of the need to urinate and once the stream starts they cannot stop it.

Some residents may have **overflow incontinence**. The person may feel as if they can never empty their bladder completely and may pass urine again right after urinating. Men with prostate problems may have this type of incontinence.

Physiological causes of incontinence

- ♦ Weakening of pelvic diaphragm

- ♦ Disorders of urethra and bladder outlet

- ♦ Disorders of bladder and surrounding tissue

- ♦ Disorders in neurological control such as spinal cord injuries.

Functions of Digestion

Mechanical - the chewing process

Chemical - enzymes present in saliva and gastric acids

Absorption - of nutrients through the small intestine

Peristalsis - a churning like motion of the bowel that moves waste

The Digestive Process

Food enters through the mouth and passes through the **esophagus** to the stomach. Digestion of food begins in the mouth but takes place mainly in the stomach. The digested food leaves the stomach and enters the small intestine. Some digestion takes place in the **small intestine**, but the main function of the small intestine is the absorption of nutrients from the food in the bloodstream. Substances which remain in the small intestine after the absorption of nutrients are waste products and fluids. They travel from the small intestine into the large intestine. The function of the **large intestine** is the absorption of fluids. Whatever remains after the absorption of nutrients and fluids, is expelled through the rectum.

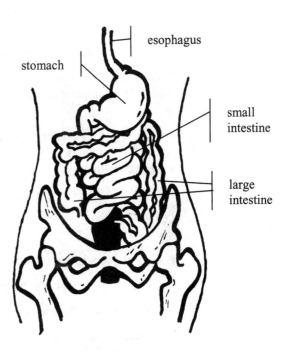

Digestive Changes Related to Aging

♦ Teeth become worn down and some are lost.

♦ There are changes in the ability to taste and smell which can affect the appetite.

♦ The esophagus may have less peristalsis. The movement (motility) of the bowel (colon) may decrease, leading to constipation.

♦ There may be loss of bowel control.

♦ There is a decrease in the secretion of the active ingredients of the saliva, leading to reduced digestion in the mouth.

♦ There is less gastric acid secreted leading to reduced digestion of food.

♦ Food is absorbed more slowly, so that older people get less benefit from the food they take in and digest

Bowel elimination means passing of waste products from the gastro intestinal system out through the rectum. The mass that is excreted is called **feces** or **stool**. This activity is also known as **defecation** or having a **bowel movement**. The frequency of a bowel movement varies from person to person. Some people have a bowel movement daily, for others a normal pattern may be every 2-3 days. Many people may have a particular time of the day that it frequently occurs. For many it's after breakfast and after consuming a hot beverage.

A normal stool is brown in color, and a soft, formed mass. Stools should be observed before being disposed.

Procedure: Assisting with the process of elimination

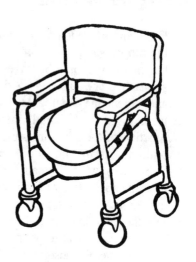

1. When there is a possibility of contact with urine or stool use standard precautions.

2. Provide for privacy and warmth of the resident.

3. Assist the resident as necessary in transferring safely onto toilet, commode or bedpan promptly as the need arises.

4. Stay close to the resident if they are unsteady, weak or confused. Remember you are responsible for their safety at all times.

5. Allow resident adequate time for defecation.

6. Leave a call light and toilet tissue within the resident's reach.

7. Position the resident in as normal a position as possible.

8. After defecation, empty the bedpan promptly.

9. Provide peri care afterwards.

10. Offer resident opportunity to wash their hands afterwards.

11. Make sure the resident is comfortable and safe.

12. Leave the call light within easy reach of resident.

13. Dispose of your gloves and wash your hands.

If you observe any of the following, save the stool and show it to your charge nurse.

dark, "tarry," black stool (this could indicate internal bleeding).

flecks of red blood in stool (possibly due to hemorrhoids)

very hard, small amounts of stool (sign of constipation)

only small smears of stool (possible sign of impaction)

presence of parasites

Common problems associated with elimination

Constipation

A frequent problem, especially with the elderly is constipation. This is the passage with difficulty of very hard, dry stool. This occurs when the stool passes through the intestine slowly, thereby getting more and more dehydrated as it remains in the bowel longer.

Contributing causes of this may be...

Inadequate fluid intake

Inadequate intake of fiber or roughage foods such as fresh fruit, fresh vegetables, whole grains, bran.

Inadequate physical activity

Lack of privacy during elimination.

Some medications and some diseases can also contribute to constipation.

Fecal impaction

If constipation is not relieved quickly enough, it could develop into **fecal impaction**. This is where the feces remains in the bowel and rectum for a prolonged period of time, getting more dehydrated and harder. The person is not able to pass it. There is a little bit of liquid feces that seeps out around the fecal blockage.

Signs and symptoms of a fecal impaction are...

Absence of normal BM for 3 days or more and

Small smears of feces only

Abdominal discomfort

Nausea and possibly vomiting

Rectal pain

Lack of appetite

If you observe these symptoms notify the nurse immediately. The charge nurse will need to take measures to relieve the impaction. The impaction needs to be taken care of promptly!

Diarrhea

Diarrhea is frequent passage of a liquidy stool. This is because the stool moves through the intestines quickly, reducing time for absorption of fluid. Sometimes diarrhea is accompanied by nausea, vomiting and abdominal pain. Diarrhea, especially in the elderly, can cause dehydration, sometimes even deadly dehydration. Report incidents of diarrhea immediately to the nurse. Provide good peri care afterwards since it can be very irritating to the skin.

Bowel Re-Training Program for Residents who are Incontinent

Starting Program

a. Elicit the cooperation and understanding of the resident. Teach and encourage resident to exercise to strengthen abdominal and other trunk muscles. Teach him the importance of an adequate fluid intake and scheduled eating time with no in between snacks.

b. Study the resident's eating habits, his physical activities, and his previous bowel evacuation pattern. Find out what the resident's usual fluid intake was and kinds and quantity of high residue foods he was accustomed to eating. Has there been a significant change in his diet and fluid intake? Inquire about his former physical activities. Was his bowel control problem preceded by a marked change in his activity pattern? Discard the concept that every resident must have a bowel movement every day. Some person's normal pattern is three to five bowel movements a week. Find out how often the resident had a bowel movement. At what time of the day did his bowel movements occur?

To Ensure Optimum Success in the Bowel Control Training Program:

a. Place the resident on a regular, eating schedule with no in between snacks. A five meal a day plan is preferable. Maintain a balanced diet for the resident.

b. Unless contraindicated medically, observe the following...

   1. Place the resident on a daily fluid intake of 2500-3000 cc. Offer fluids on an hourly schedule during the day. Be sure resident drinks three cups of fluid with breakfast every day. Encourage the resident to drink a hot beverage for breakfast.

   2. Provide a high residue diet for the resident.

   3. Give the resident 2-4 ounces of prune juice before breakfast daily until bowel evacuation pattern is established.

   4. Provide opportunity for ambulation or weight bearing daily and encourage exercises to strengthen the abdominal and other trunk muscles. These often improve bowel function.

c. Provide suitable access to toilet facilities. Wheel chair residents may need to be trained in transfer techniques.

d. Provide privacy for the resident when he is on the commode or bedpan.

e. Establish a regular scheduled time for bowel evacuation for the resident, usually about a half hour after breakfast.

Initiate the Bowel Control Program in the Morning:

a. Give the resident 2-4 ounces of prune juice orally before breakfast

b. Provide a hot beverage, such as coffee or tea, with breakfast. Encourage resident to drink 3 glasses of fluid with breakfast daily, unless contraindicated medically.

Colostomy & Ileostomy

You may have a resident who has had a colostomy or ileostomy. For a variety of reasons, whether it is due to cancer, trauma (such as bullet, stab wound or blunt injury) or bowel diseases a person may have had part of their bowel removed. The remaining part of the bowel is brought through the abdominal wall and an artificial opening (stoma) is made. Feces is now passed out through the stoma, no longer through the anus. In the **colostomy**, part of the colon is removed, in the **ileostomy** part of the ileus (small bowel) is removed. In both, the waste material is expelled through the **stoma** (exterior opening) and into a disposable plastic bag (also known as an **appliance**) applied over the stoma. The waste product can be semi-formed or very liquidy, depending on how much of the colon still remains for absorption of the fluids.

The resident is susceptible to skin irritation around the stoma site so requires excellent skin care. There are special procedures you may be taught in emptying and changing the ostomy bags.

Performing Ostomy Care

1. Remove the ostomy appliance that is attached to the skin.

2. Cleanse the area around the stoma with soap and water. Dry the area thoroughly.

3. Apply skin protector around the stoma.

4. Empty the collection bag and observe the consistency, color and amount of stool.

5. Apply the appliance and fasten the clamp.

6. Observe and report any irritated, red or open area around the stoma or complaints of discomfort.

Chapter 14 - Quiz Yourself

True or False

1. _____ All residents, once incontinent, will be incontinent for the rest of their lives.

2. _____ To help a female resident empty their bladder completely, it is important to have them sitting upright.

3. _____ Fracture bed pans are smaller bedpans for residents who cannot move or bend much.

4. _____ A resident with diarrhea may easily become dehydrated.

5. _____ Every person must have a bowel movement every day.

6. _____ Black, "tarry" stool could mean the resident is bleeding internally.

7. _____ Incontinence is an inevitable part of aging for everyone.

8. _____ Residents with Alzheimer disease may also be incontinent.

9. _____ If a resident is incontinent, you should limit their fluid intake.

10. _____ Providing privacy at toileting time is not important.

Match the term to the correct definition

11. void _____

12. meatus _____

13. urethra _____

14. defecate _____

15. commode _____

a. to have a bowel movement

b. to pass urine

c. exterior opening to urinary tract

d. a tube through which urine flows from bladder to exterior opening

e. portable bedside toilet

Circle the one correct answer

16. When doing pericare it is important to wipe...

   a. from front to back.
   b. from back to front.
   c. either of the above.

17. A resident with an indwelling urinary catheter should have the following minimum daily intake.

   a. 1000 cc
   b. 1600 cc
   c. 2000 cc
   d. 2500 cc

18. My main function is to absorb nutrients.

   a. liver
   b. small intestine
   c. large intestine
   d. stomach

19. Which are NOT digestive changes associated with aging?

   a. less peristalsis in the esophagus
   b. less gastric acid secreted
   c. large intestine absorbs fluids
   d. food is absorbed more slowly

20. The urinary catheter drainage bag should be...

   a. above the level of the catheter and bladder
   b. below the level of the catheter and bladder
   c. it does not matter

21. What is the difference between constipation and impaction?

   _____

   _____

Chapter 15
The Resident's Environment

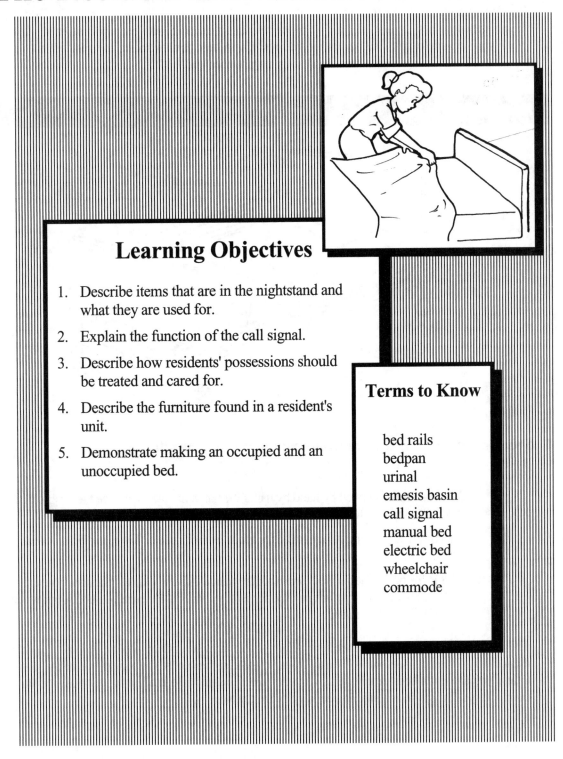

Learning Objectives

1. Describe items that are in the nightstand and what they are used for.

2. Explain the function of the call signal.

3. Describe how residents' possessions should be treated and cared for.

4. Describe the furniture found in a resident's unit.

5. Demonstrate making an occupied and an unoccupied bed.

Terms to Know

bed rails
bedpan
urinal
emesis basin
call signal
manual bed
electric bed
wheelchair
commode

The Resident's Personal Space

All caregivers need to remember that the resident's room is their personal, private space. When you enter their room you are entering their "home" and are handling their personal possessions. Conduct yourself as if you are a visitor in their home. Handle their belongings carefully and follow the resident's wishes. When taking care of the resident make them the center of the care. That is, work your schedule and routine around the resident rather than working the resident into your schedule. Their wishes and desires should be paramount to you.

The Resident's Unit

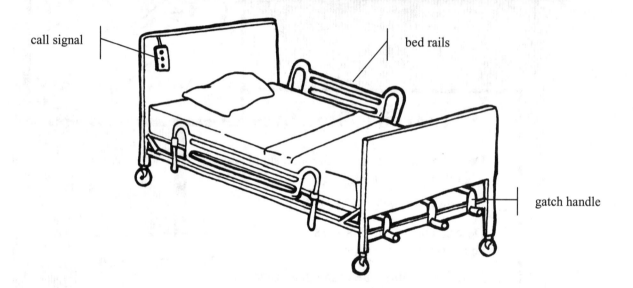

The resident's unit has the following equipment and furniture.

1. The bed

    a.) **Manual Bed**- operated by hand by using the gatch handle to change the position of the bed. Be sure to fold the gatch or crank out of the way to prevent injuries.

    b.) **Electric Bed**- the control can raise the entire bed or raise or lower the head or the foot of the bed.

    c.) **Bed Rails** on the Bed- Used to protect the resident from falling. They are considered a type of restraint so may not be used for every resident. Be sure you check out when or if bed rails are to be used.

The bed has wheels that lock. Make sure before you transfer a resident into the bed that the wheels are locked so the bed does not roll away from you. Keep the bed at the lowest horizontal position unless you are at the bedside providing care. At that time, elevate the horizontal position so it is comfortable for you in maintaining good body mechanics.

2. Overbed Table- This may be used to serve resident's meals or for treatments or personal care. Remember this is to be a clean area so do not put anything dirty such as soiled linen or equipment on the overbed table. Clean the overbed table at least several times a day.

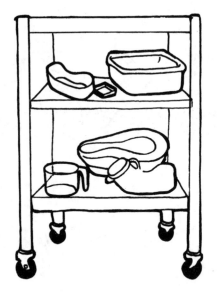

**Bedside
Stand**

3. Bedside Stand- This is used for storage of personal care items such as...

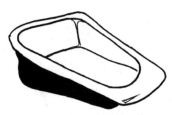

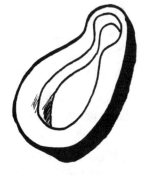

   a.) **bedpans**- used for passing stool/bowel movements for those who cannot get out of bed.

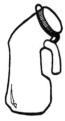

   b.) **urinals**- a container that males urinate into if they are not able to get to the toilet. Bedpans and urinals are stored on the bottom shelf of the night stand, separate from "clean" items like wash basins.

c.) **emesis basin**- a kidney shaped pan into
which a resident can spit up vomitus or
emesis, or can be used while brushing
teeth for spitting water into.

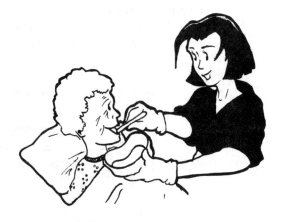

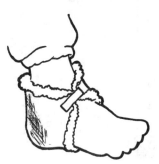

d.) special equipment such as splints, hand rolls, heel
protectors, etc.

e.) daily care items such as toothpaste, toothbrush,
mouthwash, dental floss, comb, brush, soap, nail
care items, lotion, kleenex, moist wipe pads,
gloves, etc. These are usually kept in the top drawer
of the nightstand.

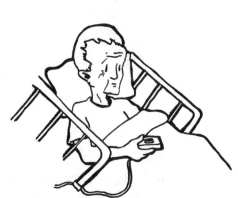

f.) water pitcher and glass for drinking are kept on the
nightstand or overbed table within easy reach of the
resident.

g.) **call signal**- be sure to leave this always
within reach of the resident so they can signal
if they need assistance. When the resident
pushes the call signal button, a light will go
on outside the room and at the nurses station.
Caregivers should respond promptly to the
call signals. There is also a call signal in the
bathroom.

Other Equipment

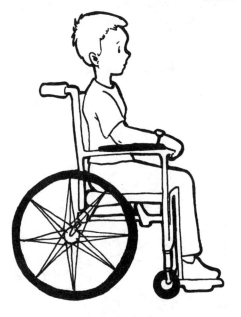

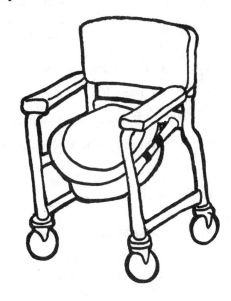

a.) **wheelchair**

b.) bedside **commode** - a movable chair that can be brought to the bedside with a removable pan that the resident can defecate (have bowel movement) into. Make sure to lock brakes in the commode wheels.

Maintaining a Pleasant Living Environment

Part of maintaining a pleasant living environment is keeping it odor free. The best way to eliminate odors is to get rid of the source. For example, promptly empty bedpans, do careful peri-care, empty emesis basins quickly, etc. Be sure to keep the resident's unit clean, neat and uncluttered. Remember that this is the resident's personal space that should be treated carefully and respectfully. Pictures, momentos and objects of sentimental value helps make this a personal and more home like living environment.

Bedmaking

The resident needs to have their bed made for them daily. A bed that is neatly made, that is clean and free of wrinkles, helps keep the resident comfortable and helps maintain good skin condition. This is particularly important for the resident who may spend a great deal of time in bed.

When the resident is able to get out of bed, you can follow the unoccupied bed procedure. There may be residents who cannot get out of bed at all and you will need to follow the occupied bed making procedure.

Before you make the bed, adjust the height of the bed to a height comfortable for you, keeping in mind rules of good body mechanics. Make all one side of the bed then complete the other side of the bed. This will help reduce wear and tear on your back. When you have made the bed be sure to lower it so the resident can get in safely.

The order in which you place the linen on the bed starting from the bottom is...

♦ Bottom sheet - flat or fitted

♦ Draw sheet if one is used for the resident.

♦ Underpads for residents who may be incontinent

♦ Top sheet

♦ Blanket

Procedure: Making an Unoccupied Bed

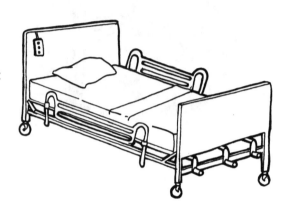

1. Assemble your supplies at the bedside: clean bottom and top sheets, blanket, pillow cases, soiled linen hamper, disposable gloves, possibly a gown, and draw sheet and incontinent pad if they are used.

2. Arrange clean linen in the order you will use them on a clean surface in the resident's room.

3. Provide for the resident's privacy throughout the procedure.

4. Lower the head of the bed so it is flat. Raise the bed to a height comfortable for you.

5. Apply gloves if the linen is wet or soiled. Use a gown if there is a risk of contaminating your uniform.

6. Remove the soiled linen by rolling it inward in a ball with the soiled or wet parts inside the ball. Dispose of soiled linen in the soiled linen hamper.

7. Remove and discard the soiled gloves and gown appropriately.

8. Wash your hands.

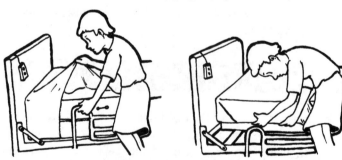

9. If using a flat bottom sheet, place the middle fold of the bottom sheet in the center of the bed and open the sheet. Place the bottom of the sheet even with the foot of the mattress. Tuck the top of the sheet even with the foot of the mattress. Tuck the top of the sheet under the mattress. Miter the corners of the top at a 45° angle perpendicular to the mattress as shown. Make sure the bottom sheet is tight and free of wrinkles. If using a fitted bottom sheet, tuck it securely over the mattress.

10. Place a draw sheet across the middle and tuck it in on the sides if it is used. Place an incontinent pad on top if one is necessary for the resident.

11. Place the top sheet with the middle fold in the center of the bed. Position the top of the sheet even with the top of the mattress. Open the sheet.

12. Place a blanket or bedspread on top.

13. Miter the top sheet and blanket or bedspread at the foot of the bed. Do so on the other side of the bed also.

14. If the resident is going to be out of the bed most of the day, make a closed bed. This is done with the top sheet and blanket pulled to the top. The spread and top sheet is turned back slightly from the top. A pillow is placed on top. The open end of the pillow should be away from the door for a neat appearance as one enters the room.

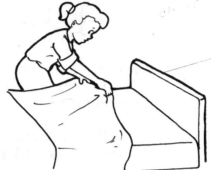

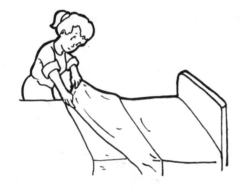

15. If the resident will be returning to the bed shortly, an open bed can be made. This is where the top sheet and spread are fan folded to the foot of the bed.

Procedure: Making an Occupied Bed

1. Assemble supplies and have ready at the bedside: clean bottom and top sheet, blanket, pillow cases, soiled linen container, disposable gloves, possibly a gown, and draw sheet and incontinent pad if they are used.

2. Place clean linen on a clean surface in resident's room. This can be a clean bedside stand, overbed table or chair. Place them in the order you will use them.

3. Provide for resident's privacy throughout the procedure. Keep the person covered while linens are changed.

4. Lower the head of the bed so the resident is lying flat in a supine position. Raise the entire bed so it is at a comfortable working height for you.

5. Apply gloves if linen is wet or soiled. Use a gown if there is a risk of contaminating your uniform.

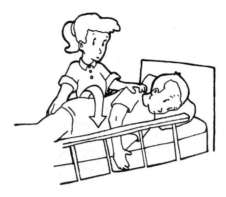

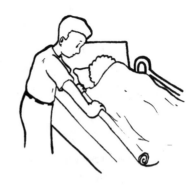

6. Loosen the top sheet. Raise side rail and roll resident toward the raised side rail.

7. Loosen soiled bottom linen and roll it toward the resident.

8. Place and tuck clean bottom linen on your working side. If a draw sheet is used, place it on top of the bottom sheet. If an incontinent pad is used, place it on top of the draw sheet.

9. Raise side rails on your side. Turn the resident toward you onto the clean linen.

10. Go to the other side of the bed and remove the soiled linen.

11. Pull and tuck in the clean linen. Make sure the bottom sheet is tucked in firmly and is free of wrinkles.

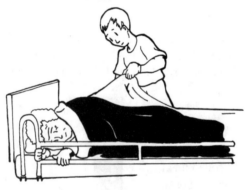

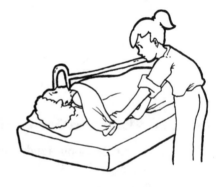

12. Cover the resident with a clean top sheet and remove the soiled top sheet.

13. Make sure the clean top sheet is centered and tucked in as necessary.

14. Replace pillow cases.

15. Avoid touching soiled linen to your clothing.

16. Lower bed to lowest height. Leave the side rails raised or lowered according to the resident's care plan.

17. Make sure the resident is safe and comfortable.

18. Dispose of soiled linen in soiled linen container. Do not put soiled linen on the floor.

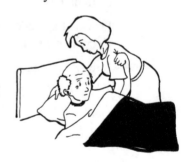

19. Discard gloves if used. Wash your hands.

When handling linen, remember infection control principles.

- Do not shake or flap linen, to avoid raising dust.

- Do not touch the linen unnecessarily.

- Do not clutch linen (clean or dirty) to your uniform.

- Use standard precautions. This includes use of gloves when there is a possibility of touching body fluids on soiled linen (urine, stool, saliva, wound drainage, etc.). Wear a gown if there is a chance of your uniform coming in contact with body fluids.

- Wash your hands before and after starting the procedure.

- Never throw dirty linen on the floor.

- Avoid having clean and dirty linen touch.

- Never place clean linen on a dirty surface.

- If you overestimate and bring too much clean linen into the room, place it in the soiled linen container. Once linen is in a resident's room, it is considered contaminated!

- Place linen that is contaminated with body fluids in a plastic bag that is secured at the top.

- Keep soiled linen hampers covered.

- Soiled and clean linen hampers must be kept separated in the hallways. Follow your facilities policy but the distance between the hampers should be at least 10 feet.

Chapter 15 - Quiz Yourself

True or False

1. _____ A bed rail is considered a restraint.

2. _____ It is acceptable to place soiled linen on the overbed table.

3. _____ The call signal must be left within reach of the resident at all times.

4. _____ Before making the bed, adjust the height so it is comfortable for you. This helps decrease strain on your back.

5. _____ When assembling your supplies for making a bed, place them in the order you will use them.

6. _____ If a resident cannot be moved from bed, the bed linen cannot be changed.

7. _____ The clean and dirty linen hamper should be kept separated by a distance of 2 feet.

8. _____ When storing items in the nightstand, be sure to keep "clean" items like wash basins separated from items considered "dirty" like bedpans. They need to be kept on separate shelves.

9. _____ The resident's bed should be made weekly.

Circle the correct answer

10. If you will be handling linen soiled with body fluids, you should...

    a. wear gloves and use standard precautions.
    b. discard it into a plastic bag tied at the top.
    c. throw it on the floor.
    d. a and b
    e. none of the above

11. Which of the following statements regarding linen handling is **false**?

    a. Wash your hands before and after handling linen.
    b. It is acceptable to shake and flap the linen.
    c. Keep soiled and clean linen hampers covered.
    d. Once linen is in the resident's room, it is considered contaminated.

12. Which of the following is a **false** statement.

    a. To insure safety while transferring, lock wheelchair and bed brakes.
    b. Toothpaste, toothbrush, and soap is usually kept in the nightstand top drawer.
    c. The best way to eliminate odors in the nursing facility is to use lots of air freshener spray.

Chapter 16
Rehabilitation and Restorative Concepts

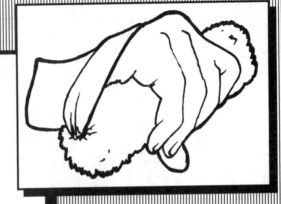

Learning Objectives

1. Describe the goal of rehabilitation.

2. Explain who the members of the rehabilitation team are and what their roles are.

3. Describe at least 3 assistive devices.

4. List at least 4 hazards of immobility.

5. Demonstrate passive range of motion.

6. Describe active range of motion exercises.

7. Describe the benefits of ROM exercises.

8. Explain what foot boards, splints, and hand rolls are and why they are beneficial.

9. Apply a hand roll.

Terms to Know

rehabilitation
rehabilitation team
assistive devices
disuse syndrome
range of motion
passive range of motion
active range of motion
foot board
splints
hand roll
contracture

Hazards of Immobility and the Disuse Syndrome

The motto for the body really is "if you don't use it you lose it". Our bodies were meant to be carried upright, walking, bending, stooping, and deep breathing. If something happens which prevents this, such as a stroke or spinal injury, complications will set in. An example of such a complication is development of a contracture in a joint that is not moved through its normal range of motion. Some complications of immobility can even be life threatening. A person who does not move much may develop pneumonia. This occurs because this person breathes shallowly which allows fluids to accumulate in the lungs which contributes to pneumonia. Another life threatening complication is development of blood clots. When a person does not move much, blood circulates sluggishly which makes it easier for blood clots to form. A clot that blocks a vessel to the heart, brain or lungs may be deadly. The following illustration details some other complications of immobility...

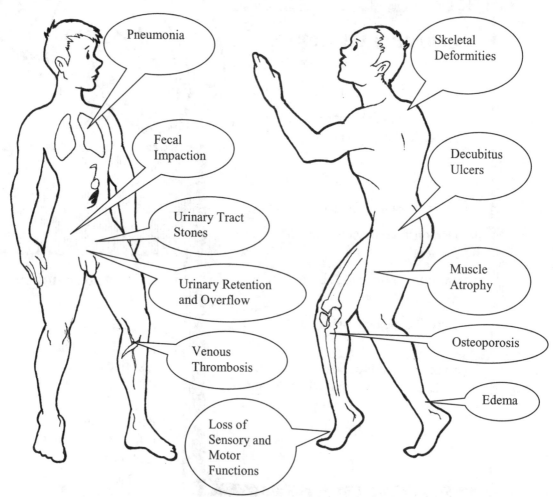

To prevent these complications, we need to keep the resident moving. This can be done by encouraging the resident to do as much for themselves as possible, such as feeding, dressing and ambulation. For residents who cannot do these skills, rehabilitation programs to re-learn skills are helpful. Range of motion exercises and good positioning is crucial also.

As human beings we feel better about ourselves and experience a higher quality of life if we can be as independent as possible. Everyone would like to take care of their own toileting, bathing, dressing and feeding. Unfortunately, due to illness or accident, this is not possible for many of our residents. They may have suffered a stroke that has left them paralyzed or experience weakness due to multiple sclerosis or had an amputation of a leg due to diabetic complications. Their previous life as they knew it has drastically changed and they are now dependent on others.

As health care givers our goals are to...

♦ prevent complications of immobility while the resident is less active. These complications can range from decubitus ulcer development to contractures to pneumonia.

♦ help the resident re-learn self-care skills such as toileting, dressing, bathing and independent feeding.

♦ return the resident to independent living at home. Unfortunately it may not be realistic for every resident to return to independent living. Some may have very severe disabilities or progressive illness that prevents this.

Rehabilitation is working toward regaining the highest level of function possible. The goal usually is to return to full function and independent living. Rehabilitation means professional skilled care provided by physical, occupational, or speech therapists to the resident.

Looking at the Whole Person

In trying to restore or rehabilitate the resident, we need to look at the whole person and provide support both physically and emotionally. The person who has lost their physical abilities may be depressed, angry, discouraged and frustrated. Activities they took for granted are now a struggle or perhaps impossible. Their world as they knew it has ended. We as caregivers, need to be sensitive, understanding, patient and encouraging. We need to stress what they are able to do and build on accomplishments. As members of the rehabilitation team we can work with the resident toward their reclaiming their independence. This process needs to start from the first day they enter the health care facility.

Adaptive/Assistive Devices

These are pieces of equipment that help the resident function more independently despite their disabilities. An occupational therapist is helpful in identifying which adaptive device is useful to the resident. They may include...

♦ special eating utensils such as a "spork" which is a combination of spoon and fork.

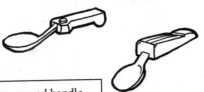

built up handle or curved handle utensils for easier gripping

food guards on plates or built up edges on plates to help residents push food against them

Chapter 16 - Rehabilitation and Restorative Concepts

♦ self dressing devices such as...

    long handled combs, sponges, shoe horns

    clothes and shoes with velcro closures

    button hookers

The Rehabilitation Team

The team is comprised of members of various health care disciplines. They are...

♦ The resident - the most important member. Their attitude, motivation and drive will help determine the outcome.

♦ The resident's family - Their support can help keep the resident motivated.

♦ The nursing assistant (NAC) - Your involvement is vital.

♦ The charge nurse (RN) - Helps coordinate rehabilitation services and assesses the resident's progress.

♦ The occupational therapist (OTR) and/or the occupational therapy assistant (COTA) - helps the resident develop strength and coordination of fine motor muscles especially of the hands. The OTR helps the resident re-learn self care and evaluates for need of assistive devices.

♦ The registered physical therapist (RPT) and/or the restorative therapy assistant works on large motor muscles to regain mobility.

♦ The speech therapist or pathologist - helps the resident regain speech and/or overcome swallowing difficulties.

♦ The physician - makes diagnosis and prescribes treatments.

Your Role On the Team

The nursing assistant plays a very important role on the team. You must...

♦ be aware of hazards of immobility and work hard to avoid them by keeping the resident as active and mobile as possible.

♦ do ROM exercises as directed by the charge nurse.

♦ be aware of when the residents have therapy sessions and have them ready and/or transport them to the therapy department.

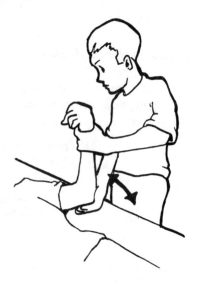

♦ be patient and encouraging.

♦ be aware of assistive devices and use them according to the care plan.

♦ participate in care meetings.

♦ observe residents for problems or progress.

♦ consult with the charge nurse if you have questions.

Restorative Nursing Care

In working toward independence, it is necessary for the resident to regain dressing, hygiene and feeding skills. Special programs such as progressive self feeding programs, hygiene and grooming, mobility and ambulation programs, work toward this goal. Read directions on the care plan for the resident and follow carefully. Carefully document the resident's progress.

ADL skill	Rehabilitation consultant	What You Need To Do...
Bathing and Hygiene	Occupational Therapist	Assist with bathing and dressing skills. Start with what they are able to do and assist with what they cannot do. Dressing adaptive devices are useful.
Self Feeding	Occupational Therapist	Assist with feeding only as necessary and encourage resident to do as much as possible. Set up trays, open containers, cut meats, etc. Adaptive self feeding devices as ordered can be beneficial.
Mobility and Ambulation	Physical Therapist	Assist with helping the resident learn to transfer from bed, move about in bed, use wheelchair, and ambulate.

Contractures

A person may not use a joint for a variety of reasons, such as paralysis, pain, being immobilized in a cast or because a person may be in a coma. If they do not move a joint through its normal range of motion, atrophy will set it. **Atrophy** is a weakening and shortening of a muscle due to lack of use. Shortly thereafter, in days or weeks, a permanent contracture may set in. A **contracture** is a shortening and tightening of the soft tissue resulting in loss of motion in the joint.

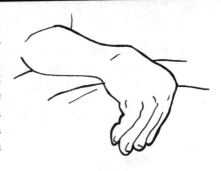

The following are contractures that may occur...

♦ hip flexion contractures - shortening of the muscles in the front of the hip, the resident will stand with the hips bent and be unable to straighten up.

♦ heel cord contracture also known as "**foot drop**". The cord at the back of the leg tightens resulting in a permanent toe-pointing downward position. The resident cannot walk on this foot.

♦ knee flexion contracture - the knee is permanently drawn up.

♦ neck flexion contracture - residents cannot lift their head up. The back becomes rounded and residents can only see out the sides since they cannot lift their head.

♦ upper extremity contractures include shoulder, elbow, wrist and finger contractures.

Contracture Prevention

Everyone on the health care team needs to work diligently to prevent contractures in the resident. Contractures can be painful, limit future positioning options and lead to permanent deformities. Hand contractures cause an inability to feed and dress oneself, prevent independence in ADL's and so much more. Knee and foot contractures rob a person of independent ambulation. These are devastating but preventable complications that can limit independence.

There are various ways we can help prevent contractures...

♦ Encourage residents to do as much for themselves as possible, if they are capable of it. Sometimes we think we can do a better and quicker job of dressing or feeding them. If we do so despite the fact that they are capable of it, we deprive them of the satisfaction of doing something for themselves and of the opportunity to move their joints. Some residents need partial assistance but can do a portion of the tasks themselves. Encourage them to do so!

♦ Use hand roll or hand splint as indicated in resident's care plan, to prevent hand and finger contractures.

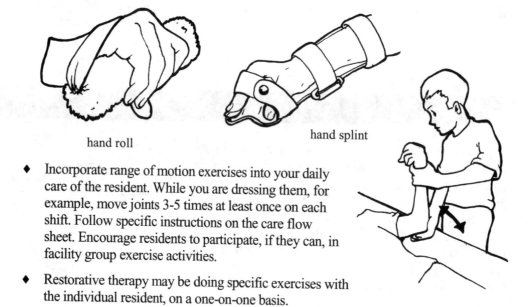

hand roll   hand splint

♦ Incorporate range of motion exercises into your daily care of the resident. While you are dressing them, for example, move joints 3-5 times at least once on each shift. Follow specific instructions on the care flow sheet. Encourage residents to participate, if they can, in facility group exercise activities.

♦ Restorative therapy may be doing specific exercises with the individual resident, on a one-on-one basis.

♦ Assist with ambulation at every opportunity possible. If they are capable of it, ambulate them to the bathroom, dining room, and activity room rather than transporting them by wheelchair. Remember, "if you don't use it, you lose it!!!"

What is Range of Motion?

A very important part of rehabilitation is maintaining range of motion. **Range of motion** is the way joints move. Residents who are not able to move and exercise normally may suffer from muscle wasting and weakening known as atrophy. This can lead to contractures resulting in a permanent deformity. Contractures are very serious complications of inactivity and limit ADL skills and independence. To prevent contractures, you need to assist with ROM exercises as directed in the care plan.

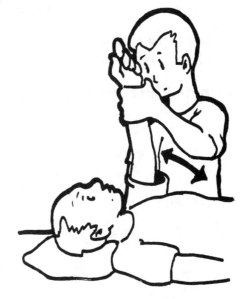

Purpose of ROM Exercises

- ◆ maintain optimum range of motion in joints
- ◆ prevent contractures
- ◆ maintain muscle strength and coordination
- ◆ stimulate circulation

Types of Residents Who Need ROM

- ◆ debilitated residents too weak to move on their own
- ◆ paralyzed residents, due to stroke, spinal cord injuries, etc.
- ◆ residents immobilized because of fractures
- ◆ comatose or semi-comatose residents
- ◆ joint damaged residents, such as due to arthritis

Points to Remember

- ◆ Never grasp belly of muscle, do support the joints.
- ◆ Tell the resident what you are about to do.
- ◆ Incorporate ROM into daily care.
- ◆ Move the limb slowly and evenly through its painless range 3-5 times.
- ◆ Watch the resident's face for indication of pain if they can't speak.
- ◆ Never force a joint!
- ◆ ROM should be performed 2-3 times daily.
- ◆ Encourage the resident to do as much of ADL's for self as possible. Continued self movement for as long as possible will keep joints limber, flexible and stronger.

- ◆ Do not do ROM to neck.
- ◆ Work systematically from top of the body to bottom, exercising both strong and weak side of body.

Types of ROM

Active range of motion (AROM) is when the resident does his own ROM. If a resident has one side paralyzed they may be able to use their non-paralyzed side to exercise their paralyzed side.

Passive range of motion (PROM) exercises are performed by the nursing assistant to maintain movement and prevent deformities.

Common Joint Movements

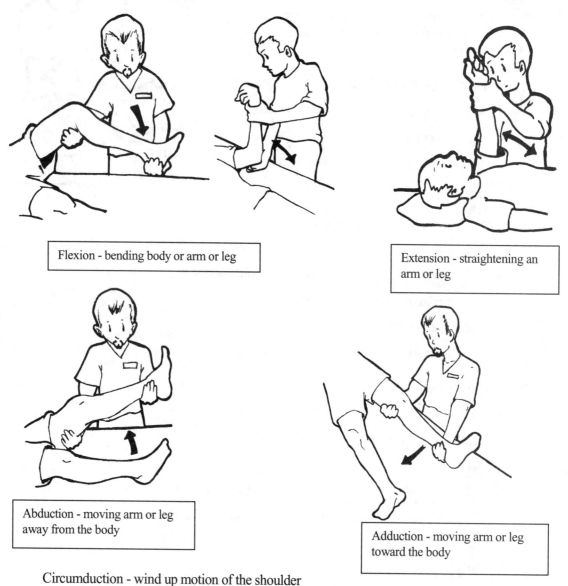

Flexion - bending body or arm or leg

Extension - straightening an arm or leg

Abduction - moving arm or leg away from the body

Adduction - moving arm or leg toward the body

Circumduction - wind up motion of the shoulder

Rotation - turning head from side to side

Doing Hand ROM Exercises

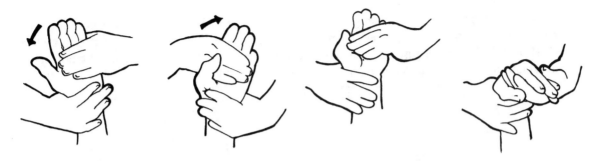

Procedure: Performing Passive Range of Motion (PROM) to one Shoulder

1. Instruct the person to inform you if pain is experienced.

2. Support the resident's arm at the elbow and wrist while performing ROM to shoulder.

3. Raise the resident's straightened arm from side position upward toward head to ear level and return arm down to side of body. This flexion and extension motion needs to be done at least 3 times.

4. All movements must be done gently, slowly and smoothly through the range of motion to the point of resistance. Observe for any indications of pain and discontinue exercise if pain occurs. Indications of pain may be verbal expression of pain, moaning or facial grimacing.

5. Move the resident's straightened arm away from the side of body to shoulder level and return to side of body at least three times.

6. Leave the bed in the lowest position.

7. Leave the signaling device within the resident's reach.

8. Wash your hands.

Procedure: Perform Passive Range of Motion (PROM) for one Knee and one Ankle

1. Instruct the person to inform you if they experience pain.

2. Support the resident's leg at the knee and ankle while doing ROM exercises.

3. Bend the knee and then return the leg flat to it's normal position. Repeat this extension and flexion motion at least 3 times.

4. Support foot and ankle close to bed while performing range of motion to ankle.

5. Keep the foot on the bed, push/pull the foot toward the head and push/pull the foot down, with toes pointing down. This is called dorsiflexion. Repeat this at least 3 times.

6. All movements must be done gently, slowly and smoothly through the range of motion to the point of resistance. Observe for indications of pain and discontinue exercise if pain occurs.

7. Lower the bed to its lowest position.

8. Leave the signaling device within reach of the resident.

9. Wash your hands.

Restorative Equipment

Splints are used to maintain good alignment by keeping the arm or leg in a fixed position. This can reverse early contractures or prevent them from occurring at all. Splints will be prescribed by the OTR or RPT. The nursing assistant should follow the care plan regarding when and for how long the splint should be worn. Before putting on the splint, check the area under the splint for redness, irritation or skin breakdown. Report any problems to the charge nurse.

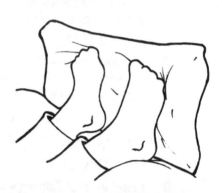

Hand rolls are used to prevent fingers from tightening into a firm contracture. The contracture can result in a tight fist that cannot be opened.

Foot boards are used to prevent foot contractures known as foot drop. Foot drop prevents a person from standing normally on their feet and causes an inability to walk. Foot boards are placed at the end of the bed. The sole of the feet should be against the foot board for support and heels hanging over the end of the mattress to prevent pressure on the heels. You can also put a pillow against the foot board and have the feet rest against the pillow.

Prosthesis

A prosthesis is an artificial body part. Prosthesis may be an artificial arm, hand, leg, foot, breast, or eye. The purpose of a prosthesis is to help the resident function as independently as possible. The resident's care plan will specify the care required including how to apply, remove, and care for the prosthesis.

The arm, hand, leg or foot prosthesis require special skin care considerations. This means checking daily for any redness, irritation, open areas or blisters on the skin under the prosthesis. If any irritation is noted, it should be promptly reported to the charge nurse. The skin under the prosthesis must be kept clean and dry. The resident usually will wear a stump sock under the prosthesis to protect the skin from the pressure of the prosthesis.

Chapter 16 - Quiz Yourself

Select the one correct answer

1. The resident is able to do his or her own ROM. This is called...

    a. passive ROM
    b. active ROM

2. Which of the following statements about ROM are **not** true?

    a. When doing ROM, stop at the point of resistance or pain.
    b. It is acceptable for the nursing assistant to do ROM to the neck of the resident.
    c. Watch for indication of pain in the resident.
    d. Do ROM 2-3 times a day.

3. Bending an arm or leg is called...

    a. flexion
    b. extension
    c. circumduction

Mrs. S. has had a stroke resulting in right sided paralysis. The concern is that she may develop contractures.

4. What can be done to prevent a hand contracture?

    _____

5. What can be done to prevent foot drop?

    _____

Mrs. S. has difficulty with bathing, dressing and feeding herself, and transferring from bed to chair. List which member of the health care team works with the resident on re-learning the following skills.

6. bathing and hygiene skills _____

7. feeding skills _____

8. ambulation and transfer skills _____

Describe an adaptive/assistive device that is helpful with...

9. self feeding _____

10. self dressing _____

11. Describe residents who would benefit from ROM exercises.

_____   _____

_____   _____

12. List at least 4 hazards of immobility

_____

_____

_____

_____

13. What can you do to minimize hazards of immobility?

_____

14. Before applying a splint, what should you check for?

_____

Chapter 17
Dementia Care

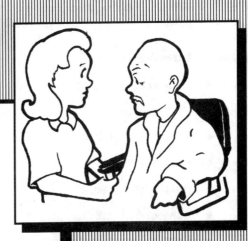

Learning Objectives

1. Define dementia, delirium and depression.

2. Describe the difference between dementia and delirium.

3. Describe what Alzheimer disease is.

4. List at least 5 behaviors a dementia resident would exhibit.

5. Describe at least 5 losses of abilities a person with dementia would have.

6. Demonstrate how to best communicate with a person who has Alzheimer's disease.

7. Describe an environment most helpful to a dementia resident.

8. Identify three potentially stressful situations a dementia resident may encounter during the day and how to de-escalate the stress.

Terms to Know

hallucinations
sundowning
manual cueing
verbal cues
dementia
Alzheimer disease
delusions
empathy
cognitive impairment
catastrophic reaction
delirium
depression

The term dementia is a broad term that covers many symptoms and many causes that can occur when the brain is damaged by disease or illness. It results in loss of cognitive function. Cognitive function includes memory, judgment, reasoning, comprehension and behavior. In dementia there is loss of brain cells and the overall size of the brain can shrink. It is not a normal part of aging. The onset is slow, it is progressive and irreversible. Many different conditions can result in dementia.

Causes of Dementia

- ◆ Alzheimer's disease (slightly more than half of all dementias)
- ◆ AIDS related dementia
- ◆ Traumatic brain injury
- ◆ Pick's disease
- ◆ Huntington's disease
- ◆ Lewy Body Dementia
- ◆ Korsakoff's syndrome
- ◆ Down's syndrome
- ◆ Crentzfeldt-Jakob disease
- ◆ Vascular dementia due to stroke (CVA) or gradual damage due to diseased blood vessels that interrupt blood flow to the brain

Common Effects of Dementia

- ◆ Memory loss, short and long term memory impairment.
- ◆ Aphasia – inability to come up with the right words, not being able to communicate needs and not being able to understand the spoken and written words.
- ◆ Not being able to follow multi-step directions.
- ◆ Not being able to recognize previously familiar people, The person may not recognize friends and relatives.
- ◆ Visual spatial changes and peripheral vision loss.
- ◆ May ask the same question over and over.
- ◆ May repeat the same story over and over.
- ◆ Loss of motor skills. This can include loss of job skills, toileting, bathing, walking, dressing etc.
- ◆ Difficulty with math.

- Inability to problem solve and learn.

- Loss in ability to control emotions and impulses.

- Inability to tell time.

- Become easily frustrated and overwhelmed. This may result in aggressive or hostile behavior. The person may strike out verbally and/or physically.

- Unable to recognize objects, sounds or images. This is called agnosia. Examples are not recognizing that a comb is for combing hair, that shoes are for wearing on feet.

- Unable to use objects properly. This is called apraxia. Examples are not using a knife for cutting food.

- Experience delusions, that is, false thinking, not based in reality. Examples are a belief that someone is stealing from them or that their spouse is not who they say they are.

- Experience hallucinations, that is, seeing or hearing something that is not real. An example is seeing a monster in the closet.

- Experience paranoia or suspiciousness. An example is that the resident may feel that someone is trying to kill them.

- Sleep pattern disturbance. The resident may sleep during the day and be awake at night or not be able to sleep at all.

- Wandering, searching or rummaging behavior.

- Tearfulness

- Depression, that is, a mood disturbance far sadder than sadness. Symptoms may include a change in sleep or appetite, fatigue, anxiety, feeling suicidal.

- Outbursts of anger

- Fearful of being alone or being abandoned.

- Catastrophic reactions, that is, an over reaction totally out of proportion to a situation. The resident may cry, scream, yell, become agitated and combative.

- Repetitive actions, such as, pacing, rocking, rubbing an object, etc.

- Resistance to care being provided. An example is not wanting to take a shower or be assisted with dressing.

- Inappropriate sexual behavior.

- "Flat Affect", facial expression or demeanor expresses little or no emotion.

- Unable to communicate needs verbally. The resident may not be able to use words appropriately or not even be able to make sounds.

Delirium

There are other conditions that may result in symptoms similar to dementia. Usually there is a rapid onset of acute confusion.

Causes of Delirium

♦ An infection, virus or inflammation. Pneumonia and urinary tract infections are examples.

♦ Medication toxicity.

♦ Electrolyte imbalance. (sodium/potassium)

♦ Malnutrition and/or dehydration.

♦ Fever or low body temperature.

♦ Anemia

♦ Thyroid problems.

♦ Liver or kidney disease.

If these conditions are treated, the dementia-like symptoms may disappear. It is critically important that a diagnosis is made so the person can get prompt treatment. Some of these causes can be life threatening so immediate medical intervention is necessary. If you notice sudden onset of confusion in your resident, report it immediately to your supervisor.

Depression

Depression is an illness that can affect anyone at any time in their life. It involves mood and thinking. Causes of depression may a response to a traumatic event such as loss of a loved one, loss of a job, loneliness, boredom, etc. or a chemical imbalance which may be hereditary. Symptoms of depression are...

♦ Loss of interest in life and activities.

♦ Low energy.

♦ Decreased appetite, possible loss of weight.

♦ Feeling sad and hopeless.

♦ Suicidal thoughts.

♦ Change in sleep, either sleeping too much or too little.

♦ Being unusually emotional, weepy or agitated.

A person with dementia may also be depressed. Depression can make dementia worse. It is important to get professional evaluation for the person so an accurate diagnosis can be made and effective treatment started. If the resident expresses any suicidal ideation (suicidal thoughts) report this immediately to your supervisor.

Environmental Factors and Dementia

Environment may be too large or cluttered- this can cause over-stimulation and cause confusion and agitation. Residents do better in a smaller environment. For example some residents function better in a small dining area with no more than 4-6 people rather than in a large, noisy dining room. Smaller units within a health care facility may be helpful.

Lack of cues from the environment- lack of clocks, calendars, newspapers, and items that orient residents as to time, date, place. These items should be placed where residents can clearly see them. Information such as the date, the season, time, and the next event coming up, should be included in your conversation with residents. This can help anchor them in the here and now. All the hallways and doors may look alike making it difficult for them to find their way. Any distinguishing feature such as a picture, momento, or special keepsake that may trigger a memory may help them recognize their room.

Over-stimulation from the environment- the health care facility may be a very noisy place with background music and TV noise, noisy roommates, hustle and bustle of the staff, that can cause a resident to get agitated. This over-stimulation can continue on a 24 hour a day basis with interrupted sleep and rest periods for the resident.

Lack of stimulation of the environment- this can pertain to the resident who is left for long periods of time in their room with no involvement in meaningful activities or socialization. The care giver also may not provide adequate stimulation if they do not make eye contact with the resident, do not explain what they are going to do and not engage the resident in conversation appropriate to their level of understanding.

Unfamiliar environment or lack of routine- it takes residents a long time to adjust to a new environment when they are first admitted. Having familiar items, furniture and pictures that resemble their home can help. Having daily routines can be reassuring to residents but it should be flexible enough to accommodate their specific needs. For example if a resident refuses a bath, see if another time would be more acceptable.

Causes related to the task- Task may be too complicated with too many steps involved. A task like dressing oneself may involve too many steps, such as picking out clothes, undressing, putting on various items of clothing. These sequential steps may be overwhelming for the resident. The resident would benefit from **verbal cueing**, that is the caregiver would assemble the supplies and talk the resident step by step through the process allowing the resident to complete the steps one by one. **Manual cueing**, that is demonstrating and starting a task can be helpful also. An example is putting toothpaste on a toothbrush and bringing it up to the resident's mouth. If a resident is unresponsive to verbal cues, put your hand on his/her hand and gently offer guidance.

Alzheimer Disease

In the U.S. 5.3 million people have **Alzheimer disease**. It is the 4th leading cause of death in the U.S.. Alzheimer disease is the major cause of irreversible mental decline in the elderly, being responsible for about 50% of such cases.

Alzheimer disease is a progressive condition that affects areas of the brain involved in making judgments, language, memory and behavior. One in eight people age 65 and older now has Alzheimer, half of those 85 and older have it. It is a progressive disease resulting in the destruction of brain cells. It's course may last 7-12 years from onset to death. This condition may vary from patient to patient with some deteriorating quicker than others.

Frequent causes of death are complications of immobility such as pneumonia. This occurs when the resident is in advanced stages of Alzheimer and has lost the ability to ambulate. Decreased mobility contributes to fluids accumulating in the lungs, leading to pneumonia and death. This occurs as the resident starts to "unlearn" things they had known before. Just as an infant and toddler learns to walk, feed themselves, dress themselves, learns words and masters language and speech, an Alzheimer patient "unlearns" these abilities. As Alzheimer's disease advances, speech, language, ambulation, ADL skills, feeding, chewing and swallowing abilities gradually are lost.

The cause of Alzheimer at this time is yet unknown. Researchers do believe that lower levels of acetylcholine, a chemical messenger (neurotransmitter) in the brain, does not allow nerve cells to work properly. It is also believed that a protein known as beta-amyloid collects between nerve cells, disrupting brain function and triggering an immune response that destroys cells. Plaques that are clumps of amyloid deposits and tangles (twisted strands of protein) disrupt the normal structure of nerve cells and are visible on examination of the brain after the person has died. Risk factors for developing Alzheimer seem to be having heart disease, diabetes, being a smoker, and having a relative with Alzheimer.

We are now at a point where researchers understand the mechanism of Alzheimer much better but there is still much more to learn. Currently there are medications to help deal with the symptoms of Alzheimer but hopefully in the near future there will be drugs to actually slow down or reverse the disease itself.

Stages of Alzheimer's Disease

Various experts break down Alzheimer disease into different stages with different characteristic behaviors. This particular approach breaks down Alzheimer into 3 stages.

Stage 1 - Mild Dementia

Early in this stage the resident may appear normal, with very subtle deterioration. The resident may be able to cover up some of the changes at first but as memory and personality changes increase, it is evident something is definitely wrong.

Symptoms and Behaviors

♦ Short term memory loss.
♦ May get lost even in familiar surroundings.
♦ Feeling anxious, agitated and depressed.
♦ Short attention span and not being able to concentrate.
♦ Lack of attention to hygiene and appearance.
♦ Feeling that someone is out to harm them.

> **What we can do!** The person may have difficulty functioning in their usual environment. They would do best in a simplified environment with reduced noise and confusion, and cues to help them such as signs, pictures and familiar objects. Verbal cues and breaking down tasks can be helpful, i.e., talking a resident through self dressing by giving them directions, one step at a time, moving slowly, giving the resident lots of time to process the information.

Stage 2 - Moderate Dementia

The behaviors of Stage 1 continue. Long term memory loss is affected now also. Resident is unable to do ADL skills independently.

Symptoms and Behaviors

♦ Wandering, pacing and restless behavior. Sundowning or increased restlessness in the late afternoon or evening becomes more of a problem.
♦ Repetitive behavior or movement such as rocking back and forth, rubbing an object, etc.
♦ Unable to recognize and avoid dangerous situations.
♦ Not able to understand and follow directions.
♦ Impulsive behavior, not thinking out consequences of behavior.
♦ Increased difficulty in communicating.
♦ Difficulty reading and writing.
♦ Catastrophic reactions.
♦ Hallucinations
♦ Delusions
♦ Stiff, shuffling gait and poor balance.
♦ Incontinence of bowel and bladder.
♦ Loss of peripheral vision and difficulty in tracking an object.

What we can do! Travel back in time to where the resident is. Concentrate on pleasant reminiscence and non-verbal communication such as hugs, touch, smiles, walking, smelling aromas, and feeling textures.

The resident can benefit from self-feeding training programs, dressing and ambulation programs. An environment with low stress, low noise and a leisurely pace is most effective. Since the resident may have poor peripheral vision remember to make sure items are in their visual field. For example, are you sure they actually see everything on their plate at mealtime?

The person will need help with ADL tasks. Provide verbal cues (talk them through what you are doing) and manual cues (demonstrate and get them started on the task). Quiet, small groups are less overwhelming to the person than large groups.

Insure safety for residents. Residents may have poor judgment and not recognize dangers or hazards. A safe environment must be provided with careful monitoring and supervision. This can include safety measures to prevent falls and burns and precautions to insure that the resident does not wander away from the facility.

Stage 3 - Severe Dementia

All previous problems continue and deteriorate further. The resident loses the ability to take care of self and is totally dependent on others.

Symptoms and Behaviors

♦ Unable to recognize loved ones.
♦ Disoriented completely as to time and place.
♦ Difficulty swallowing with increased risk of aspiration.
♦ Unable to communicate needs.
♦ Unable to walk.
♦ Resident loses weight and is unable to regain it.
♦ Resident is susceptible to lung and bladder infections.

> **What we can do!** Maintain a safe, quiet, gentle environment. Do not rush the resident. Provide comfort, keeping them clean, dry and turned every 2 hours. Soft, soothing music, hugs and touch are helpful. Reassure resident that they are safe and loved. Provide plenty of fluids and snacks if their diet permits.

How to Deal with Behavioral Disturbances

Some people suffer from **hallucinations**. This means seeing, hearing or feeling something that is not real. An example is seeing animals, people or other objects which may be scary. Others may have **illusions**. This is when they misinterpret objects. For example, they may misinterpret the bush outside their window as a bear. Some residents may suffer from **delusions** which are false beliefs. Examples are believing they are someone famous, like a movie star, thinking someone is out to murder them or thinking that a loved one is really someone else.

The best way to handle the above behaviors is **not** to argue with the resident and not to convince them that they are wrong. What they believe is very real to them. Instead, if they are fearful, be calm, reassuring them that you will protect them. Additionally re-directing them to some activity or distracting with some object may help. Remember that these behaviors are part of the disease process and something the resident cannot control.

Many residents become more stressed, are more agitated and have more difficulty coping in the late afternoon and early evening. This is called **sundowning**. It is good to provide rest, a calm environment, and snacks at this time. Hunger can add to restlessness. Do not put demands or expectations on the resident.

Wandering, rummaging behavior, and pacing - The resident may have a seemingly uncontrollable urge to keep moving. There are several things you need to do, including reassuring them that they are safe. Make sure that they are in an alarmed area that would keep them secure and away from streets, traffic, etc. Do not try to reason with the person but use distraction to re-direct them if necessary. Residents may respond well to doing repetitive simple tasks such as folding towels instead. Additionally, mark their door with a personal, identifiable object to help them recognize their room.

Catastrophic reactions are over-reactions that are out of proportion to the situation. Residents cannot control their behavior. They may become agitated, restless, possibly aggressive and even violent. They may yell and scream. Catastrophic reactions are in response to situations that feel overwhelming to them. They may feel that they have no control over their life. The best approach is to prevent catastrophic reactions from occurring by observing what seems to trigger them and avoiding those situations. When a catastrophic reaction occurs, do not argue with residents. Speak to them in a quiet, calm reassuring manner. Distract, re-direct and gently remove them from the stressful situation or environment. Do not restrain or use physical force. Stand to the side and out of reach of residents if there are safety concerns. Get help if needed but avoid overwhelming them with too many people.

Inappropriate sexual behavior – Some behaviors you may witness are mistaken for sexually inappropriate behavior. A resident who is wandering in a public area without clothing is not necessarily an exhibitionist but does not remember to dress. Residents who touch their genital area may have pain or irritation related to UTI, impaction, yeast or vaginal infections. Residents who get in bed with someone may do this because of their disorientation rather than sexual desire.

A small group of residents, however, may engage in sexually inappropriate behavior like public masturbation, fondling, inappropriate touching or actual attempts at intercourse. These behaviors should be immediately reported to the charge nurse. The risk of the resident harming others must be evaluated carefully and a plan developed. An unconsenting resident must be protected from a sexually aggressive resident.

Aggressive Behavior - Anger may be an emotional response to feeling fear, frustration, or loss of self-esteem. Additionally, certain stressors such as hygiene activities, especially showers, getting out of a cozy warm bed, being awakened early in the morning, a noisy environment, over crowded and over stimulating situations can trigger an angry response. Residents can express their anger verbally or physically by becoming agitated and/or combative. Ideally we can identify possible causes of aggressive behavior and work toward defusing the situation before it escalates.

Possible causes of aggressive behavior

- ♦ feeling little control over daily decisions
- ♦ loss of freedom of choice in daily activities
- ♦ inability to communicate effectively
- ♦ lack of privacy
- ♦ physical discomfort
- ♦ illness
- ♦ fear of something that is not understood
- ♦ fatigue

Ways to prevent and/or de-escalate agitated or aggressive behavior

- ♦ develop a trust relationship with the resident. Do not make any promises you can not keep.

- ♦ explain what you are doing and identify yourself to the resident

- ♦ offer choices and decision making opportunities

- ♦ speak in a calm, clear manner, give simple directions and watch for feed back

- ♦ use distraction to refocus residents who become agitated

- ♦ do not rush residents, allow them to set the pace

- ♦ anticipate residents' needs

- ♦ prevent fatigue

- ♦ respect their personal space and belongings

- ♦ provide for privacy

- ♦ acknowledge feelings residents may have. If they appear angry, you might say "I can see that you are angry". Listen carefully to residents and try to help resolve the situation.

- ♦ treat residents with respect and courtesy

Anything we can do to minimize stresses in a resident's life may make them feel more calm, happy and improve orientation.

Assisting with meals

The environment should be uncluttered and quiet. Small, non-noisy dining rooms are easier for the resident as compared to large stimuli filled dining rooms. In a quiet dining room the resident is less likely to be distracted and can concentrate on verbal cues regarding eating. Praise and smiles from the caregiver improves resident self esteem. Offering residents 1 to 2 items on their tray at one time is less confusing, as opposed to 6 items all at once. Do not rush residents!

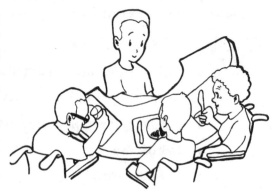

Communicating with the resident

A person with dementia may have difficulty understanding words so non-verbal communication is even more important. Approach the person from the front or slightly to the side, at their eye level so you do not appear to be looming over them or threatening in any way. Appear calm, friendly and unrushed with a smile on your face. Introduce yourself, call them by their name and tell them what you are about to do. Speak slowly and clearly. Give simple one or two step directions. Avoid negative words like "don't" but phrase it by saying "Let's walk down the hall . . . etc." Encourage and praise your residents so they feel good rather than focusing on their disabilities such as memory loss.

It is helpful to communicate an idea to residents utilizing as many senses as possible. For example, before bathing residents, let them smell the soap, touch the soap, water and towel, hear you use words like "bath," "clean," "wash", see the bathing supplies and clean clothes. These various senses help residents get the idea. When residents are prepared and understand the activity, they are more likely to be relaxed and cooperative. When residents are exhibiting negative behaviors the most effective approach is to...

- ◆ ignore the behavior

- ◆ re-direct or distract residents with some other activity

The person may not be able to communicate effectively with words but listen to, recognize and respond to their emotions. Do they appear to be upset, frightened or frustrated? Be patient and respectful in your communication. Do not use words like "remember?", "I told you that already". They do not remember so do not ask them questions that make them feel inadequate. Continue to communicate with residents at their level and allow them to express their wishes. Communicate in a way that is supportive and helpful to the person. Listen to what they are saying and be supportive of the emotions they are feeling. Although we do not encourage false beliefs, we encourage them to explore these beliefs. For example, a person may state "I must leave right now for my job as a teacher. My students are waiting for me". An appropriate response might be "Tell me about your job as a teacher", or "Tell me about your class". Do not argue with the person or dispute facts since this can isolate them, cause frustration and withdrawal.

Promoting Success

The environment and residents' days should be set up so residents feel successful. An example would be encouraging residents to do parts of tasks they can do without difficulty and then quietly assisting them with the rest. Praise them for their success. The caregiver should express satisfaction to residents with smiles and touch.

Recognizing the Resident's Feelings

The caregiver needs to be empathetic to the feelings of residents. **Empathy** in this case means putting yourself into their position to understand how they might feel. It builds trust and restores dignity.

When residents expresses feelings, the caregiver needs to acknowledge these feelings.. The caregiver lets residents set the pace and the tone, never being judgmental. If residents have certain feelings these are valid feelings. The caregiver should never argue, reason or try to convince them of something they do not believe.

Homework

What can you do in the following situations?

1. Mr. Thompson, a mildly confused gentleman, is extremely upset when you enter his room today. What are you going to say to him?

   A. "What is the matter? Can I help in any way?"

   B. "It's a wonderful day today, Mr. Thompson. What would you like to do today?"

   C. "Now, now, Mr. Thompson, things can't be that bad. If you think you have problems, listen to mine..."

2. Mr. Johnson, who was just admitted, has been incontinent three times on your shift. You do not yet know the nature of his problem. What would be the appropriate thing to say to him?

   A. "You really must make some effort to stay dry."

   B. "Don't worry about it. I'm used to cleaning up after everyone here."

   C. "I'm sorry this happened. I imagine you feel embarrassed about this. Let's see what we can do so this doesn't happen to you again. I will check with you every 2 hours and take you to the bathroom."

3. Mrs. B. is an 88 year old lady who was recently admitted. Her husband who took care of her at their home died 6 months ago. Mrs. B. paces a lot during the day, cries and tries to leave to find her home. She has difficulty dressing herself and doing her own ADL's. She has difficulty finding her room.

   Name three things we can do to help Mrs. B. settle in, make her feel at home and orient her to her new surroundings.

   _____

   _____

   _____

4. Mrs. Smith is an 87 year old woman who cannot get out of bed, get dressed or ambulate on her own. She is confused as to where she is and strongly insists that you get her to her school. She explains that she is a teacher and that her children are waiting for her. What can you say to Mrs. Smith?

   _____

   _____

   _____

True or False

1. _____ Alzheimer is one of the leading causes of death in the U.S.

2. _____ When a resident has hallucinations or delusions, argue with them and point out that they are wrong.

3. _____ If a person is experiencing a catastrophic reaction, restrain them.

4. _____ An environment that is quiet, calm and reassuring is helpful to the agitated resident.

5. _____ Delusions are false beliefs.

6. _____ One difference between delirium and dementia is that the onset of delirium is acute and sudden.

7. _____ Cognitive impairment means a decrease in intellectual functioning such as reasoning, thinking and memory.

8. _____ Do not offer any choices to the dementia resident.

9. _____ Loud television can help calm the restless, agitated resident.

10. _____ An Alzheimer disease resident may not recognize their family members or know how old they themselves are.

Multiple Choice (circle the one correct answer)

11. Sundowning means

    a. The resident is agitated when they awaken at night.
    b. The resident has exaggerated dementia symptoms in late afternoon and early evening.
    c. The resident has delusion symptoms on dark, cloudy days.

12. Alzheimer disease may result in which of the following problems?

    a. diarrhea
    b. incontinence
    c. loss of ability to ambulate
    d. none of the above
    e. b & c

13. Which of the following are NOT symptoms or behaviors of advanced Alzheimer disease?

    a. tearfulness
    b. inability to communicate needs verbally
    c. sleep disturbances
    d. pain in toes

14. Which of the following is not a cause of dementia?

    a. AIDS
    b. Alzheimer disease
    c. Down's syndrome
    d. pneumonia
    e. Pick's disease

Chapter 18

Death, Dying, and Grieving

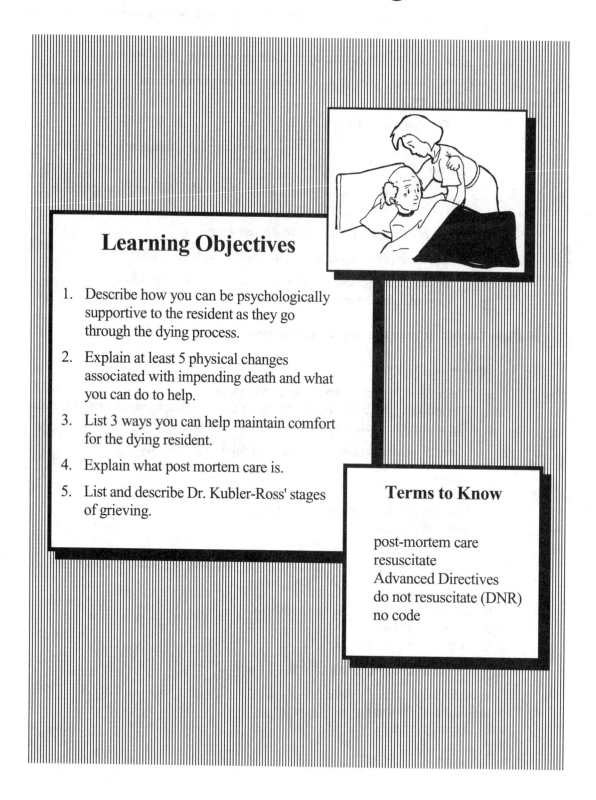

Learning Objectives

1. Describe how you can be psychologically supportive to the resident as they go through the dying process.

2. Explain at least 5 physical changes associated with impending death and what you can do to help.

3. List 3 ways you can help maintain comfort for the dying resident.

4. Explain what post mortem care is.

5. List and describe Dr. Kubler-Ross' stages of grieving.

Terms to Know

post-mortem care
resuscitate
Advanced Directives
do not resuscitate (DNR)
no code

As a nursing assistant you will have occasions to take care of terminally ill residents and take care of the body of a resident who has died. You will also need to deal with grieving families and friends. You need to know what to do and how to do it but also understand what your feelings are pertaining to death.

Our feelings and attitudes about death, which are shaped by our religion, culture and previous experiences, affect how we take care of people. Recent studies of caregivers in hospitals showed that they actually on many occasions spent less time with the dying resident. This may be because they are uncomfortable with the whole issue of death, may feel that they may not be able to change the likely outcome (death) or may be fearful that they may not say the "right thing." Whatever the reason, the end result can be that the resident does not get the physical and emotionally supportive care they deserve.

In order to provide good, competent nursing care you need to know yourself! You need to examine your feelings about death. You can do this by talking to your supervisor, your clergy person or doing some reading on this topic. This is crucially important because the care you provide to your dying resident may be influenced by your attitudes. If you are uncomfortable about death, you may not be comfortable in listening to the resident who may want to tell you what they are feeling. Your discomfort may deprive them of this important opportunity for support.

The resident and their family have spiritual and emotional needs. As caregivers you need to be respectful of the spiritual belief system of the resident even if it is not yours or if you do not agree with it. Be courteous to the clergy and the resident's religious customs, rituals and religious objects. Do not impose your religious beliefs on the resident.

Stages of Grief

The dying resident has emotional, psychological and physical changes and needs as they approach death. Dr. Elizabeth Kubler-Ross has written several books on this topic. In her book, "On Death & Dying", she details the grieving that the resident and their family may go through. In her observation and work with many dying people, Dr. Kubler-Ross saw that these stages and behaviors were very common in most people. Not everyone will go through every stage, sometimes they may advance through the stages and then move backwards. Everyone is different and the length of time in each stage may vary. Ideally the resident will work their way to the acceptance stage where they are more at peace with their situation. The resident's loved ones go through these stages also. Be sensitive and supportive of their needs.

Steps of the Grieving Process

1. **Denial** - The person cannot believe, absorb or accept that this is happening to them. This is the temporarily protective mechanism until the person can have this information sink in. In this stage the person denies that death may be an imminent possibility. Do not try to convince them, instead listen sympathetically.

2. **Anger** - The person may be angry at the world, including family and caregivers. They may be argumentative, combative, demanding and unpleasant. Do not take this behavior personally but try to see how it fits into the overall picture.

3. **Bargaining** - This is more of an internal process in the resident that you may not see externally. Depending on their belief system the person may bargain with God for more time. An example may be "God, if you let me live until the birth of my first great grandchild I will be a better person." That is, asking for something from God and offering something in return.

4. **Depression** - Signs of depression may be weepiness, crying, withdrawn behavior, not wanting to get out of bed, not getting dressed, not sleeping, not eating, lack of eye contact. The best approach for the caregiver is to be gentle, caring and encouraging, and being available to the resident if they want to express their feelings but not forcing conversation. A resident is more likely to express their feelings if they are comfortable with you and have a trust relationship established. If they know they can trust and rely on you they may open up and unburden their feelings. This is very helpful to the resident. The most important thing the caregiver can do is to be a good listener. Do not worry so much about saying the "right" thing. Do not give false reassurances to the resident.

5. **Acceptance** - The person realizes and accepts their situation. They are more at peace and may make plans such as wills, giving away items of sentimental value, etc.

Do Not Resuscitate

When a resident is admitted the physician and charge nurse need to explore with the resident what their wishes are regarding end of life issues. The resident may possibly sign a **"Do Not Resuscitate" (DNR)** or **"No Code"** order. This means the resident does not wish to have CPR or extraordinary means to resuscitate them. To **resuscitate** means to revive or bring back to life, if there is an absence of vital signs. The resident may also have **"Advanced Directives"** signed. These are pre-written instructions on what life prolonging measures the resident may want if any. It is the resident's life and it is their decision regarding these important issues. If the resident is incapable of making these decisions, their legal guardian can make these decisions for them.

Maintaining Comfort

Depending on the nature of their terminal illness, the resident may suffer from pain and discomfort. Residents, especially in their final weeks and days, deserve to be as comfortable as possible. We are getting better at controlling pain with improved medication. It is up to the health care team to observe the resident and make sure that they are comfortable. As the nursing assistant you should observe for any indications that a resident is in pain. This can include...

- ♦ Complaints of pain

- ♦ Non-verbal expressions such as grimacing, holding or favoring one part of the body.

- ♦ Crying and/or moaning

Report instances of pain to the charge nurse who will insure that the resident receives the prescribed medications. You may be asked to document instances and severity of pain. If the current pain management regime is inadequate, the charge nurse will consult with the physician who may prescribe a different medication, dosage, or pain management approach.

The nursing assistant needs to work at keeping the resident as comfortable as possible by...

- ♦ Good positioning. This includes changing position at least every 2 hours and using supportive positioning devices such as pillows.

- Making sure the resident is clean and dry with fresh, non-wrinkled linen.

- Giving a back rub to help relaxation.

- Insuring comfortable room temperature. If the resident is cold due to decreased circulation, add warm blankets and socks.

- Positioning a short of breath resident in a Fowler's position.

- Leaving call signal within reach of the resident and responding promptly to the needs of the resident. This can help decrease fear and anxiety over being left alone and make the resident feel secure that someone is there to respond to them when needed. When a resident is less anxious they become less tense which helps them relax and feel more comfortable.

Possible Signs of Approaching Death

In the final stage of the dying process, the body starts to shut down. This includes a slowing down of the circulatory system, including decrease of oxygen to the brain and internal organs and decrease of circulation to extremities. There will be changes in metabolism and the level of consciousness. These gradual physical changes are normal, natural and to be expected. The body is preparing for all physical systems to stop functioning. The best thing we can do is to insure that the resident is kept as comfortable as possible through this process.

The last sense to be lost as a person approaches death is hearing. Although a person may appear to be sleeping or appear unconscious they may hear and understand. Never say anything in the presence of a person that you would not want to be heard.

The Following are Signs of Approaching Death

What you may see...   What you can do...

What you may see...	What you can do...
The resident becomes weaker with decreased strength, endurance and flaccid (limp) muscles.	Assist the resident with ADL tasks such as dressing, hygiene, toileting, turning and positioning. Make sure to turn them at least every 2 hours for comfort and good skin care. Back rubs frequently can be very helpful.
The resident will feel cool or even cold to the touch, especially in the hands and feet. The extremities may also have a grayish-bluish color. Circulation to the extremities is starting to decrease. The resident feels cold.	Keep the resident covered with extra blankets to keep them warm. Put warm socks on feet. Keep hands covered. Increase the room temperature if needed to keep the resident comfortable.
A change in the breathing pattern may occur. There may be noisy congested sounding respiration (gurgling sounds). The resident may not have the strength to cough up secretions from the lungs. Respirations may be rapid, shallow and panting. A change in regularity of breathing may occur including Cheyne-Stokes breathing. This is when there is an absence of breathing for 5-30 seconds followed by normal breathing.	Elevate the head of the bed into a Semi-Fowler's position. Turn the resident's head to the side to allow gravity to drain the secretions. Due to general weakness, the resident may not be able to cough up and clear their own secretions.
The person may become incontinent of urine and/or stool.	Keep the resident clean and dry. Check for dryness at least every 2 hours.

The Following are Signs of Approaching Death (cont.)

What you may see...   What you can do...

The person may be confused and disoriented as to time, date, and place. They may not recognize loved ones. They may be sleeping more and more and lapse into periods of unresponsiveness.	Remember that a resident may be able to hear and understand even if they are unresponsive. Say only what you want them to hear in their presence. When entering the room, identify yourself and explain what you are about to do. Identify people in their presence to them. Be reassuring and supportive.
The person may get restless, anxious and make repetitive movements such as, pulling at their clothing, or calling out.	Maintain a calm, soothing environment and demeanor in interacting with the person. Be responsive to the resident's need. Soothing music may be helpful.
The person may want little or no food or fluids and/or have difficulty swallowing. Their lips may be dry and cracked and the tongue have a thick coating, due to lack of fluids.	Do not try to force food or fluids or nag them into eating or drinking. Small chips of ice may be refreshing on the lips. Maintain intake and output record as directed. Check with the charge nurse regarding nutritional and fluids issues. Fluids that have thickeners in them or thicker juices like apricot nectar, are easier to swallow for those that have swallowing difficulties. Oral care, including use of lemon-glycerin swabs at least every 2 hours is necessary for people who cannot swallow and/or are unconscious.
The person may tell you about things or people that they see but you do not. They may see people who have already died. This is a common occurrence. It may be calming to the resident or disturbing to them.	Do not argue with the resident, or try to convince them that what they saw is unreal or contradict what they see. Be available to the resident if they wish to talk about their fears and concerns.

Changes after Death

- ◆ Jaw will drop
- ◆ Pupils are fixed and dilated
- ◆ Body gradually loses heat and becomes cool
- ◆ Muscles relax so resident may pass urine, feces or flatus (gas)
- ◆ The body stiffens (rigor mortis) within 6-8 hours
- ◆ Very pale skin color

Postmortem Care

Postmortem care refers to care of the body after death. If you are taking care of the resident when they die you will also be responsible for post mortem care. The resident's family may come to view the body before they are removed to the mortuary. It is important to make sure the resident is neat & clean and presentable. Each facility may have their own specific post mortem care procedure.

When providing post mortem care be sure to treat the resident's body with respect and dignity just as you did when they were alive. Pull privacy curtains and do not expose any parts of body to others view.

Procedure: Post Mortem Care

1. Assemble your supplies. Use gloves and standard precautions as appropriate.

2. Pull curtains for privacy. Place the body in a supine position.

3. Close the eyes. If the eyelids do not remain shut, apply a moistened cotton ball on each eye lid.

4. Follow facility policy regarding dentures.

5. Close the mouth with a towel under the chin to keep the mouth closed.

6. Bathe the body. Remove any soiled dressings and apply clean dressings.

7. Put on a clean gown.

8. Comb the hair. Shave if necessary.

9. Cover the body up to the shoulders with a clean sheet.

10. Check with your facility policy as to what you need to do with jewelry, glasses, hearing aids.

11. Make sure the resident care unit is neat, clean and tidy. Remove unnecessary equipment and supplies.

12. Remove gloves. Wash your hands.

Chapter 18 – Quiz Yourself

True or False

1. _____ All residents go through the stages of grieving in the same manner and at the same rate.

2. _____ All residents will reach the acceptance stage of the grieving process.

3. _____ As people near death, their circulation to extremities may decrease. They may feel cold, especially in their hands and feet.

Explain what the following terms mean

4. DNR_____

5. Advanced Directives_____

   _____

6. Resuscitate_____

   _____

7. Post Mortem Care_____

   _____

8. Describe 3 things you can do to help the dying resident maintain comfort.

   _____

   _____

   _____

Chapter 19
Special Care and Procedures

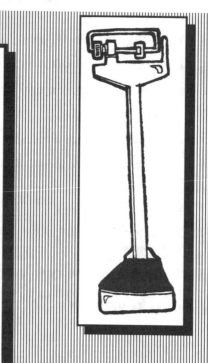

Learning Objectives

1. List the type of specimens a nursing assistant may collect.

2. Understand why specimens may be helpful as diagnostic tools.

3. Explain how stool specimens are obtained.

4. Collect a sputum specimen.

5. Label specimens properly.

6. List at least 3 precautions for care of a resident with oxygen.

7. Demonstrate how to obtain a height and weight of a resident.

8. Demonstrate application of anti-embolism stockings.

9. Explain at least 3 special needs a resident in a cast may have.

Terms to Know

specimen
urinalysis (UA)
urine culture and sensitivity (C&S)
clean catch or mid-stream urine specimen
anti-embolism, compression stockings
24 hour urine specimen
sputum specimen
stool specimen
dyspnea

A nursing assistant may be responsible for obtaining specimens which may be a valuable diagnostic tool. A specimen is a sample of material taken from the resident's body. Specimens include urine, feces, and sputum specimens.

Urine Specimens

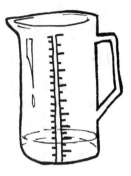

Urine is a source of much information to the physician about the resident, including whether there is an infection and whether there is a problem with the urinary system. This valuable information can help the physician diagnose a problem or evaluate current treatment. This is done by obtaining a **urine specimen (sample)** and sending it to the laboratory for study. The urine specimen is sent for a **urinalysis (UA),** meaning an analysis or study.

A **urine culture and sensitivity (C&S)** is a test to check what kind of pathogen is present in the urine and which antibiotics will kill it. This is done in the laboratory.

As a nursing assistant you may be responsible for obtaining a urine specimen. The physician will specify what type of specimen is required of the following...

Clean catch or midstream specimen- The objective is to get a clean specimen. Prior to obtaining the specimen, clean the perineal area well with either soap and water or a designated periwash. This is important so that any organic matter is not present that would contaminate the specimen and alter the test results. The urinary stream is started, which flushes off some microorganisms and then the specimen cup is put in place to catch the remaining urine. Collect at least 100 cc's.

Routine or Random Specimen- Have the resident urinate into either the bedpan, commode or urinal. In the bathroom or dirty utility room, pour the urine from the bedpan, commode or urinal into the specimen cup.

24 Hour Urine Specimen- All urine voided during a 24 hour period of time is collected. It is started with the first voiding being discarded and all subsequent specimens collected. The starting time is labeled. The resident can void into the bedpan, commode or urinal. There should be no BM or toilet paper in the same receptacle at the same time. Empty the specimen using a funnel into the designated 24 hour receptacle that may be stored in a refrigerator. Save all the urine during the 24 hour period. Have the resident void at the end of the period. Label carefully and take the specimen to the charge nurse.

Sterile specimen- This will be done by the licensed nurse who catheterizes the resident (inserting a sterile straight catheter into the bladder) and obtaining a sterile specimen of urine.

Stool Specimen- The physician may order a stool specimen that you may need to obtain and that will be sent to the laboratory for study. When obtaining the stool specimen make sure that the resident does not urinate into the commode. If they usually defecate into the toilet, a specimen pan can be put under the seat to catch the stool into a container. Use a tongue blade to transfer about 2 tbsp. of stool to the specimen container. Fill the specimen cup half full. Label the container, put it in a plastic bag and deliver it to your charge nurse. Be sure to use standard precautions throughout this procedure.

Sputum Specimen- You may need to obtain a sputum specimen. **Sputum** is the substance that is coughed from the lungs (expectorated). Have the resident spit up into a specimen cup. Label the specimen. Be sure to wear gloves.

Label specimens accurately!

It is important that the specimens be labeled correctly. This requires the resident's name, date, and time the specimen was obtained. Print clearly and attach the label securely to the container.

- ◆ Be sure to use gloves and use standard precautions when handling specimens.

- ◆ Label the specimen with the resident's name and room number

- ◆ Do not touch inside the specimen cup or inside the lid.

- ◆ Dispose of contaminated equipment or supplies in biohazardous waste container.

Special Care

The physician may order **anti-embolism or compression stockings** for residents with edema. These stockings are also known by their brand names of TED or Jobst stockings. They apply equal pressure on the veins of the legs to promote blood flow back to the heart. This improved circulation helps prevent edema and possibly prevent formation of a blood clot. Some hose are open toe, others closed toe, some are below the knee and others above the knee. They are usually put on in the morning while the resident is still in bed, and removed before bedtime. Follow directions of the nurse however for the specifics regarding the particular resident. Before putting on the elastic hose, inspect the resident's skin, bathe and thoroughly dry between the toes and on the legs and feet. There are different sizes of elastic hose ranging from small to extra large. The appropriate size should be used. The hose should be hand washed every evening and left to drip dry. Check the temperature and color of the toes every hour. Report to the charge nurse if the toes are cool or bluish in color or if the resident complains of discomfort.

Procedure: Applying Anti-Embolism Stockings

1. Provide for resident's privacy.

2. Have the resident in a supine position while applying stocking.

3. Turn the stocking inside out.

4. Place the foot of the stocking over the foot, heel, and leg, stretching it carefully.

5. Pull the top of the stocking over the foot, heel and leg.

6. Move the foot and leg gently.

7. Make sure there are no wrinkles or twists and that the stocking is on straight.

8. Leave the signaling device within reach of the resident.

9. Wash your hands.

Obtaining Resident's Weight

Keeping track of a resident's weight can provide some valuable information. Weight changes can provide insight into nutritional status, whether there is significant fluid retention and other significant factors. What the resident's weight is can determine possible treatments or necessary dietary changes. Accurately obtaining a resident's weight therefore is an important responsibility for the nursing assistant.

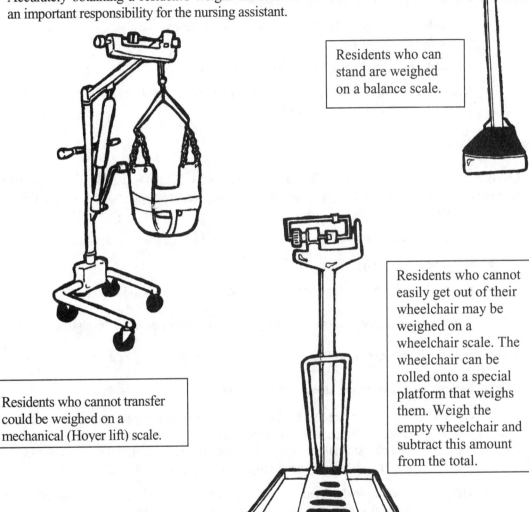

Residents who can stand are weighed on a balance scale.

Residents who cannot transfer could be weighed on a mechanical (Hoyer lift) scale.

Residents who cannot easily get out of their wheelchair may be weighed on a wheelchair scale. The wheelchair can be rolled onto a special platform that weighs them. Weigh the empty wheelchair and subtract this amount from the total.

Procedure: Obtaining a Weight of an Ambulatory Resident

1. Weigh the resident at approximately the same time of the day wearing about the same weight of clothing.

2. Make sure the resident has shoes on before walking to scale.

3. Start with the scale balanced at zero.

4. Have the resident take off their shoes and stand on a paper towel on the scale. Assist the resident to step up onto the center of the scale.

5. Balance the scale by making the balance bar level. This is done by moving the small and large weight indicators until the bar balances. Determine the resident's weight.

6. Help the resident off the scale and into their shoes.

7. Write down the weight.

Procedure: Measuring the Resident's Height

1. While the resident is on the standing balance scale, extend the height measurement rod to above the resident's head.

2. Lower the rod until it rests flat on the resident's head.

3. Record the height in feet and inches. Convert the inches into feet and inches by dividing it by 12 (there are 12 inches in a foot).

Use of Oxygen

Oxygen is vital to human life. Some illnesses can affect how oxygen is used by the body, and will necessitate administration of oxygen. The physician may order oxygen for the resident and will specify the following...

♦ method of administration (mask, nasal cannula or prongs, nasal catheter)

♦ rate (flow rate of oxygen)

♦ length of administration (period of time the oxygen is to be administered)

Oxygen may be dispensed by oxygen tank, oxygen concentrator or piped in through wall units.

The charge nurse is responsible for beginning, discontinuing, or adjusting the flow rate of oxygen.

Things the nursing assistant should remember...

♦ Oxygen is drying to the nose and mouth. If the resident has oxygen delivered by nasal prongs, good skin care around the nose (nares) is necessary. If the resident has oxygen delivered by face mask, make sure the face mask is clean and placed securely in place. Provide good skin care to the cheeks and around the ears.

♦ The resident may have **dyspnea** which is difficult or labored breathing. This can make the resident fearful and anxious. Be supportive and reassure them that you will check on them frequently. Leave the call light within easy reach of the resident.

♦ Position the resident with dyspnea in a Fowler's position which makes breathing easier

♦ Check for pressure on the skin or discomfort caused by the oxygen mask, nasal cannula or nasal catheter, and readjust as needed for comfort.

♦ Pace physical activities for residents since their strength and endurance may be limited and they may be dizzy. Assist them as needed. When transferring residents who may be dizzy, bring them up to a supported sitting position first and support them to a standing position. Allow rest periods as needed.

♦ Residents may be diaphoretic which means they may perspire heavily and their skin may feel moist. They will need frequent bed baths, sponge baths, back rubs and clothing changes for comfort.

♦ Oxygen is quite combustible. No smoking materials should be in the room, which includes, cigarettes, matches, and lighters. A "No Smoking" sign should be placed in the room and on the door to the room. Electrical equipment that may produce sparks should not be in the room.

♦ Standard precautions should be used at all times when you come in contact with body fluids such as saliva, sputum, nasal discharge.

Special Needs for the Resident with a Cast

You may be taking care of residents who may have a cast. Skin care is a special consideration since casts potentially can cause pressure at certain points.

♦ Observe for signs of impaired circulation to the limb in the cast. Watch for fingertips or toes that are cool or cold to the touch, bluish or purple in color, or swollen. Report these findings immediately to the charge nurse.

♦ Report to the nurse if the resident complains of pain or discomfort, tingling or numbness in the limb that is in the cast.

♦ Report to the nurse if the cast is wet or has an odor, or if there is any drainage from inside the cast that stains it.

♦ Keep the limb that is in the cast, elevated on a pillow.

Chapter 19 - Quiz Yourself

True or False

1. _____ The nursing assistant is the person who obtains a sterile urine specimen.

2. _____ Sputum is the substance that is coughed up from the lungs.

3. _____ It is acceptable to touch the inside of the specimen cups and lids.

4. _____ Any resident who cannot stand independently cannot be weighed.

5. _____ Another name for prescribed elastic hose is TED hose.

Circle the correct answer

6. If a resident is 64 inches in height, this is the same as...

   a. 5 ft. 4 in.
   b. 5 ft. 2 in.
   c. 5 ft. 7 in.
   d. 6 ft.

7. The purpose of a mid stream method of obtaining a urine specimen is to...

   a. obtain just a small amount of urine
   b. obtain as clean a specimen as possible
   c. obtain a sterile specimen
   d. provide another opportunity for you to wear gloves

8. Dyspnea means...

   a. difficulty swallowing
   b. weight loss
   c. swelling
   d. difficulty in breathing

Fill in the correct answers

9. Mrs. Benson broke her arm which is now in a cast. What 3 things do you need to observe regarding the cast?

   _____

   _____

   _____

10. Mrs. Bailey has been short of breath and now has oxygen administered by nasal cannula. She is anxious, dizzy and weak. Describe 3 things you need to do for her.

   _____

   _____

   _____

Chapter 20

Common Health Problems

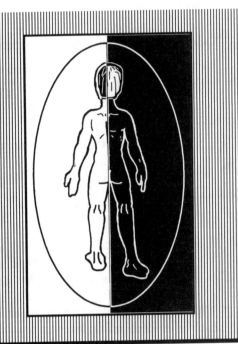

Learning Objectives

1. Describe at least 3 symptoms of CHF, COPD, and CVA.

2. List at least 3 symptoms of a TIA.

3. Explain what the possible disabilities may be when a resident has right hemiplegia and left hemiplegia due to a CVA.

4. Explain what the nursing assistant can do to help take care of a resident who has... CHF, diabetes, and COPD.

5. List at least 3 complications that can occur due to diabetes.

6. Describe at least 3 warning signs of diabetes.

7. Explain what rehabilitation services can be helpful to the resident who has had a CVA.

8. Explain what osteoporosis is and how it contributes to falls.

9. Describe what a nursing assistant should do if a resident has a seizure.

Terms to Know

seizure
congestive heart failure (CHF)
chronic obstructive pulmonary disease (COPD)
pneumonia
diabetes mellitus
transient ischemic attack (TIA)
cerebrovascular accident (CVA)
hemiplegia
one sided neglect
bronchitis
emphysema
aphasia
dysphagia
osteoporosis

Seizures

A seizure is an abnormality in the activity of the brain due to abnormal electrical discharges. It can occur from the time of birth, due to a brain tumor, head injury, abnormality in the brain chemistry or due to a stroke.

There are different types of seizures...

1. **generalized tonic, clonic seizure or grand mal**- there will be stiffness and jerking of muscles in the entire body and loss of consciousness and incontinence of bowel and bladder. This type of seizure may last several minutes. Afterward the resident may feel very tired, have a headache, be slightly confused and have slurred speech.

2. **partial small seizure or petite mal** - there may be quivering of muscles, and the resident may have change in level of alertness. This may include staring blindly or stopping what the resident is doing. This usually lasts a few minutes.

3. **simple partial (Jacksonian)** - muscle spasms start in an arm or leg and progressively moves up on that side of the body.

4. **status epilepticus** - series of seizures that continue with no breaks in between. This may occur due to infections, fever or sudden withdrawal of anti-seizure medications. This is dangerous and can lead to death.

Responsibilities of the nursing assistant during the seizure involve protecting the resident from injury and maintaining an open airway. This would include...

♦ moving the resident to a safe lying position

♦ moving something soft, like a pillow under the head

♦ moving anything hard or sharp away from the resident such as furniture, equipment etc.

♦ **NOT** restraining or inhibiting resident's movement

♦ turning the head of the resident to the side allowing for drainage of vomitus or saliva

♦ **NEVER** putting anything into the mouth of the resident

♦ while the resident is having a seizure, stay with the resident and signal the charge nurse for help. Report observations made to the charge nurse.

♦ after the contraction stage is over, tilt the resident's head back to insure an open airway.

Osteoporosis

Osteoporosis is a loss of calcium from the bones with reduced amounts of normal bone tissue. This makes the bones brittle and very susceptible to fractures. If one could see the bones affected by osteoporosis you would see that they look like a honey comb or sponge and actually weigh less than a normal bone. A person with severe osteoporosis could suffer a fracture even without an injury, possibly sustaining a fracture just by rolling over in bed or just by normal walking. This is a problem that affects millions of people. Frequently people consider this only a problem affecting women over the age of menopause but in reality over a million American men are affected also. This is a serious problem that contributes to injuries, fractures and decreased independence for many people.

There are certain factors that put a person at added risk of osteoporosis...

- Lack of activity, being immobile
- Loss of sex hormones for women after menopause
- Alcohol and smoking reduces bone mass
- Certain medications like steroids increase bone loss
- Caffeine use increases loss of calcium

Congestive Heart Failure (CHF)

Congestive heart failure is when the heart is not able to pump blood effectively. Blood backs up and results in congestion of tissues.

Residents with congestive heart failure can be treated with medications that help the pumping efficiency of the heart and diuretics that help rid the body of excess fluids. A diet low in salt is important. Ultimately congestive heart failure can result in death.

What Happens in the body with Congestive Heart Failure?

- blood does not pump efficiently causing blood to back up in the veins.
- fluids accumulate in the body, especially in the feet and ankles. This fluid retention is called edema.
- fluids can build up in the lungs called pulmonary or respiratory congestion. This can cause dyspnea (difficulty breathing), increased sputum production, cough and gurgling sound in lungs.
- circulation is inadequate to the brain causing fainting, dizziness and confusion.
- decreased circulation to kidneys causes decreased kidney function and reduced urinary output.
- finger tips and sometimes lips may be cyanotic (bluish in color due to reduced oxygen) and extremities may feel cold.

What Can You do to Help?

- pace activities according to resident's capabilities. They may need frequent rest breaks.
- position resident in semi-Fowler's or Fowler's position for easier breathing.
- follow nursing orders regarding maintaining I & O, daily weights if ordered and wearing elastic hose if prescribed.
- follow any ordered dietary restrictions since resident will probably be on a low sodium diet.
- report change of condition to the charge nurse.
- keep resident warm since their extremities (hands & feet) tend to feel cold due to poor circulation.

What is it?

Diabetes is a disease that affects the way your body turns food into fuel or energy. When a person has diabetes one of two things goes wrong, either the body does not produce enough insulin or the body cannot use it effectively. Insulin, which is a hormone produced by the pancreas helps glucose enter the cells. When glucose is inside the cells, glucose changes into energy. Diabetes has serious implications for the person because it can also affect other organs such as the kidneys, blood vessels and eyes. This occurs because the extra glucose that cannot enter the cells builds up in the bloodstream and this high blood sugar can cause damage to the organs mentioned.

Complications are Killers

Diabetes is a leading cause of death by disease in the US. Thirteen million Americans have diabetes mellitus. There are many complications that can develop.

Diabetic Complications include...

- blindness- diabetic eye disease or retinopathy is the number one cause of blindness in people under the age of 75.

- amputations- 40% of amputations occur to the diabetic because of diabetic neuropathy (nerve damage in the feet) and poor circulation to the feet and legs.

- heart and blood vessel disease- people with diabetes are 2 to 4 times more likely to develop heart disease and 5 times more likely to have a CVA (cerebrovascular accident or stroke).

- kidney disease- 32% of kidney failure cases are due to diabetes.

There are different types of diabetes

Insulin-dependent diabetes (type I) fortunately affects only 5% of the people with diabetes. It has its onset early in life, in children and teenagers. The person needs to take daily injections of insulin, and during the long course of their disease is more likely to develop serious complications.

Non-insulin-dependent diabetes (type II) affects 95% of the people with diabetes and usually occurs in adults over the age of 40. Fortunately it can usually be controlled by a diabetic diet and exercise. Some may require oral medications or insulin injections.

People who are more prone to diabetes are...

- those with a family history of diabetes

- those over the age of 40

- those that are overweight

- people of the following ethnic backgrounds: African Americans, Native Americans and Hispanics.

How Do I Know If I Have Diabetes?

The warning signs are...

- excessive thirst
- extreme hunger
- frequent urination
- weakness, fatigue, irritability
- blurred vision or vision change

- slow healing of cuts, especially on feet
- tingling or numbness in legs, feet or fingers
- frequent infections

Hypoglycemia / Hyperglycemia

When a person has diabetes they may have extremes in blood glucose (sugar) level. An excessively high amount of glucose in the blood is called hyperglycemia. An excessively low amount of glucose in the blood is called hypoglycemia. Either one of these conditions could possibly lead to coma and death. As a nursing assistant you need to observe and report any of the following signs immediately to your charge nurse.

hyperglycemia - speech may be slurred, skin may be hot, person may become confused, pulse may be slow and breath may have a sweet, fruity odor.

hypoglycemia - skin may be cold and clammy, pulse may be rapid and weak, respirations may be shallow and the person may be irritable and confused.

What Can You Do to Help Your Diabetic Resident?

Know which of your residents has diabetes so you can take special precautions such as listed below.

Do not trim the toenails of your diabetic residents - this should be done by a podiatrist or licensed nurse.

Observe special foot care precautions as detailed in the chapter on foot care.

Keep feet warm and covered.

Watch for cuts, sores or wounds on feet and report to charge nurse.

Encourage the resident to stick to the prescribed diabetic diet.

If your resident does not eat their meal well or vomits, notify your charge nurse. This may affect the insulin they may normally be given by the nurse.

Encourage movement and exercise as this stimulates circulation and keeps extremities healthier.

Notify the nurse if the resident complains of vision changes such as blurry vision, pain in their eyes, seeing double, etc.

Observe for signs and symptoms of hypoglycemia and hyperglycemia and notify your charge nurse immediately.

Chronic Obstructive Pulmonary Disease (COPD)

COPD refers to people with bronchitis and/or emphysema. This is the most common chronic lung disease and affects 15.8 million people in the US.

What is bronchitis?

This condition is inflammation of the bronchi. Bronchi are delicate tubes in the lungs that are attached to the trachea and carry air to smaller tubes in the lungs. The person may have a chronic cough, frequently coughing up mucus, pus and possibly blood. The patient may tire easily due to impaired air flow and inadequate oxygen intake.

What is emphysema?

This is a condition where the alveoli become enlarged. Alveoli are air sacs where oxygen from the air is exchanged for carbon dioxide in the blood. Alveoli do not expand and contract normally with each respiration, so air remains trapped in the alveoli during expiration. As the disease progresses more and more alveoli are involved and oxygen and carbon dioxide are not exchanged properly. Symptoms include coughing and shortness of breath, weight loss, fatigue and anxiety due to difficulty breathing. The patient becomes short of breath upon exertion and as the disease progresses even at rest.

What can the health care worker do to help the resident with COPD?

- Pace activities The resident tires very easily and will need frequent breaks to catch their breath and rest.

- Position resident in Fowler's or Semi-Fowler's position when they are especially short of breath.

- A position especially helpful is sitting up and leaning slightly forward. They may be more comfortable leaning forward onto a pillow placed on an overbed table in front of them.

- Watch for signs and symptoms of a respiratory infection such as elevated temperature, listlessness, or noisy and congested sounding respirations. Report this to your charge nurse.

Pneumonia

Pneumonia is a very serious and potentially fatal respiratory condition. It is the sixth leading cause of death, resulting in up to 70,000 people losing their lives annually. People more likely to suffer complications of pneumonia are...

- over the age of 65

- suffer from chronic conditions like asthma, emphysema, heart disease or kidney disease.

- suffer from a compromised immune system due to AIDS or chemotherapy.

- immobile, allowing fluids to accumulate in the lungs

- have aspirated fluids into their lungs.

There are different types of pneumonia

viral pneumonia - symptoms include fever, chills, weakness, loss of appetite, body aches, dry cough, sore throat, headaches, increasing breathlessness. It is usually treatable with bed rest and fluids.

bacterial pneumonia - symptoms include severe pain in the chest, sweats, productive cough with greenish mucus, cyanotic lips due to decreased oxygen, fever, chills, weakness, loss of appetite, body aches, dry cough, sore throat. Antibiotics are required to treat this type of pneumonia.

mycoplasma (also known as walking pneumonia) - This type seems to have characteristics of both bacterial and viral pneumonia. Symptoms include persistent cough that produces white mucus, fever, chills, weakness, loss of appetite, body aches, dry cough and sore throat. Antibiotics are used as treatment.

It is very important for the nursing assistant to be observant for the above symptoms and promptly report them to the charge nurse. It may be a matter of life and death! The nurse or physician will listen to the lungs, order a chest x-ray and perform blood or sputum culture to determine the cause. This will determine the course of the treatment appropriate for the resident. Prompt treatment may save the life of the resident.

Cancer

Cancer is caused by malignant cells that grow, multiply and invade healthy tissue. Malignant tumors can occur in various organs and metastasize (spread) to other parts of the body.

Treatment

- ◆ Surgery – removal of tumor and/or abnormal cells.

- ◆ Chemo therapy – medications that kill cancer cells.

- ◆ Radiation – x-ray treatment that kills tumor cells.

Special care needs

- ◆ Emotional, psychological, and spiritual – The resident may be fearful about the cancer, treatment and the future outcome. The resident may be depressed or anxious. They will need emotional support and encouragement. A spiritual advisor may be of assistance to the resident.

- ◆ Possible pain and discomfort related to progression of disease and/or side effects of treatment – Utilize comfort measures to decrease pain.

- ◆ Weakness – The resident may need assistance with ADL tasks.

- ◆ Possible decreased appetite and poor nutritional level – Monitor the resident's intake, offer small, frequent meals and foods that they can tolerate. Consult with the charge nurse and dietitian regarding nutritional supplements.

A CVA is also known as a stroke or brain attack. Cerebro means brain, vascular means blood vessel, so this means an occurrence or "accident" in the blood vessel of the brain. CVA is the third leading cause of death of people in the United States. It occurs when there is an interruption of blood supply to the brain resulting in brain damage or death. It may occur due to...

♦ a rupture of a blood vessel in the brain or

♦ a clot may block the blood from passing through the blood vessel.

When a CVA occurs, the amount and kind of disability depends on where in the brain the damage happened. Different parts of the brain are responsible for different functions so the type of disability is determined by the location involved. If the damage has occurred in the left side of the brain, weakness will appear on the right side of the body. This weakness is called **hemiplegia**. If the damage has occurred in the right side if the brain, weakness will appear on the left side of the body.

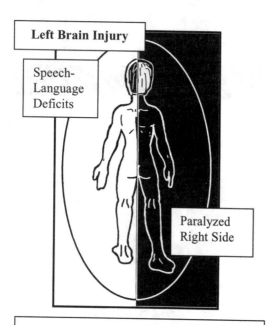

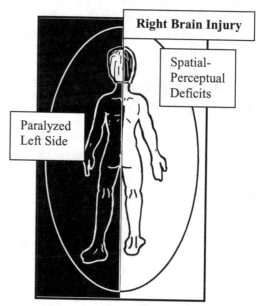

A left brain injury will result in right hemiplegia. People with **right hemiplegia** (right sided weakness) will likely have problems with aphasia. Some people may have difficulty with both speaking and communicating. Others may understand but have difficulty speaking. Read Chapter 3 on aphasia.

A right brain injury will result in left hemiplegia People with **left hemiplegia** (left sided weakness) may have difficulty with spatial-perceptual deficits. This means they may not be able to judge distance or perceive themselves and objects in space correctly. Since we cannot view the world through the resident's eyes we may not recognize how much of a problem this truly is for them. This can severely impact the residents ability to take care of themselves and affect their safety.

Spatial - perceptual deficits may manifest themselves by...

♦ difficulty knowing when the resident is leaning, sitting or standing

- not being able to steer their wheelchair through a doorway without hitting the door jam

- wheeling themselves too close to an open stair case

- missing the table when setting down a hot cup of coffee and spilling it on themselves

- not being able to visually follow columns or lines in a book or newspaper

- not being able to button all buttons without missing or skipping some.

People with left hemiplegia are more likely to have what we call **one sided neglect**. That is, they may ignore their impaired side and not perceive their body as a complete whole unit. This may manifest itself in the following ways...

- the person may not recognize his or her arm or leg as being their own. They may say "whose arm is that on my lap?"

- they may leave food on their plate on the impaired side. They may not complete their meal because they don't see, not because they are no longer hungry.

- the person may ignore or not see people, objects or activities on their impaired side.

What Happens When A Person Has A CVA?

When a person has a CVA they may experience one or more of the following disabilities...

- weakness or paralysis (right or left hemiplegia)

- dysphagia - (difficulty swallowing making the resident susceptible to deadly aspiration)

- aphasia - there may be different types of aphasia

    expressive aphasia - resident has difficulty expressing themselves verbally

    receptive aphasia - difficulty understanding what is said or what they read

    expressive or receptive aphasia - some residents have both of the above

- labile moods - uncontrollable emotional expression or over-reaction to events or stimuli. The person may frequently cry but this is not necessarily related to sadness or depression

- vision changes - there may be "visual field cuts" such as parts of the picture missing or loss of peripheral vision (what normally one can see out of the corner of their eyes)

- memory deficits - the resident may have short retention span meaning they may remember for a very short time only. They also are more likely to remember events prior to their stroke as compared to what has happened since.

- depression, anger, frustration - all understandable feelings in response to the sudden and devastating losses a person has suffered.

Is there hope for recovery?

Rehabilitation services such as physical, occupational and speech therapy are very important if the resident will regain any or all of their losses. Therapy needs to start immediately after a CVA since most improvement is likely to occur in the first six months. It can be a slow, demanding process that can leave the resident frustrated and exhausted. It is important to be supportive, encouraging and understanding to the resident as they work hard to overcome their disabilities.

Ways You Can Help

♦ Do not isolate the resident. Remember there are ways to communicate other than with words, such as pantomime, demonstrations, notepad and pencil, pictures, communication board, gestures, smiles, etc.

♦ Check the level of understanding of the resident. Do not over or underestimate their abilities.

♦ Simplify communication by speaking in a clear, concise manner but never "talking down" to the resident

♦ Break directions into simple one or two steps and give immediate feedback.

♦ Be encouraging, patient and non-critical.

♦ Keep messages simple

♦ Provide a rich stimulating environment but not over-stimulating or overwhelming to the resident with too much noise or confusion.

♦ Turn the plate of food 180^0 degrees midway through the meal for the residents with one-sided neglect. This enables them to see all the food on their plate.

♦ Approach the resident from their non-impaired side of body.

♦ Assist resident to change position at least every two hours.

♦ Watch for and prevent pressure areas.

♦ Support the resident with postural supports if needed while sitting, to prevent slumping to one side.

♦ Position properly in a supported, upright position at mealtime to prevent aspiration.

♦ Assist with daily care activities as needed.

Transient Ischemic Attacks, What are they?

Prior to a stroke, some residents may suffer a **transient ischemic attack** (TIA) which is a temporary interruption of blood to the brain. One or more of these symptoms may last only a few minutes and the patient recovers. It is important to recognize these symptoms because TIA's could be a warning sign of a possible impending stroke. Prompt medical attention may prevent a deadly or debilitating stroke from occurring. Signs and symptoms of TIA are one or more of the following:

♦ sudden weakness in an arm, hand or leg

♦ severe headache

♦ difficulty understanding what is said

♦ difficulty speaking

♦ lack of sensation on one side of the body

♦ inability to see out of one eye

True or False

1. _____ While a person is having a seizure, put something into their mouth to keep it open.

2. _____ Osteoporosis only affects women.

3. _____ Residents with CHF have edema and dyspnea.

4. _____ Stroke residents may have vision impairments.

5. _____ Symptoms of pneumonia that should be reported to the charge nurse are fever, chills, productive cough and weakness.

6. _____ If a resident has right hemiplegia, it means they are paralyzed on their right side.

7. _____ The disabilities a person suffers after a stroke depends on where in the brain damage occurs.

8. _____ A transient ischemic attack is a warning sign of a heart attack.

9. _____ After a stroke, it is important for therapy to start immediately.

10. _____ A resident who has had one-sided neglect may ignore, not be aware of or be non-protective of their paralyzed side.

Circle the one correct answer

11. Warning signs of diabetes are...

    a. excessive thirst
    b. frequently feeling hungry
    c. a & b
    d. none of the above

12. COPD refers to...

    a. bronchitis
    b. emphysema
    c. a & b
    d. none of the above

13. Another name for a stroke is...

    a. brain attack
    b. cerebrovascular accident
    c. a & b
    d. none of the above

14. List 3 possible complications of diabetes.

    _____

    _____

    _____

15. List 3 problems a stroke resident may have and what you can do to help.

    Problem   Ways to Help

    _____   _____

    _____   _____

    _____   _____

    _____   _____

    _____   _____

    _____   _____

True or False

1. _____ Average recommended fluid intake per day is 1000 cc.

2. _____ The resident has the right to refuse to take a bath.

3. _____ A TIA may be a warning sign of a stroke.

4. _____ It is alright to throw soiled linen on the floor.

5. _____ If a resident is having a seizure, force a wash cloth into their mouth.

6. _____ It is acceptable to put a dirty glove on the overbed table.

7. _____ Alzheimer disease is considered a terminal disease. A frequent cause of death is pneumonia.

8. _____ You should wear gloves when shaving a resident.

9. _____ A graduate is a measuring device.

10. _____ It is acceptable to leave dentures wrapped in a paper towel on the nightstand.

11. _____ A BP of 90/50 would be considered hypotension.

12. _____ You should carefully trim the toenails of a diabetic resident.

13. _____ Restraints can be deadly.

14. _____ If a resident is incontinent, it is highly unlikely that they will ever be continent.

15. _____ Signs of a UTI are pain on urination, and urine that is dark and cloudy.

16. _____ If you have a positive TB skin test it means that you have active infectious disease.

17. _____ There is a vaccine available and recommended for HBV.

18. _____ Symptoms of delirium are not reversible.

19. _____ Alzheimer disease residents are likely to be incontinent in their later stages.

20. _____ Do not tell a resident that you will be counting their respirations.

21. _____ A verbal cue is talking a resident through a procedure.

22. _____ If you made an error on the resident's medical record, use "white out" to mask out the mistake.

23. _____ We know that unconscious residents cannot hear or understand what is said around them.

24. _____ Position a resident who is eating in an upright position to avoid aspiration which can be deadly.

25. _____ The longest and strongest muscles are in the thighs and should be used during lifting and transferring.

Match the following terms (on the left side) to the definitions (on the right side).

26. _____ dysphagia   a. difficulty speaking

27. _____ decubitus ulcer   b. inhale into the lungs

28. _____ aphasia   c. difficulty swallowing

29. _____ aspiration   d. pressure area

30. _____ hemiplegia   a. paralysis from the neck down

31. _____ quadriplegia   b. paralysis from the waist down

32. _____ paraplegia   c. difficulty breathing

33. _____ dyspnea   d. paralysis of half of the body (vertically)

34. _____ NPO   a. stroke

35. _____ DNR   b. measurement of fluid

36. _____ CVA   c. do not start CPR

37. _____ cc.   d. nothing by mouth

38. _____ abdominal thrusts   a. unable to pass stool due to blockage

39. _____ impaction   b. sample

40. _____ constipation   c. passing hard stool

41. _____ specimen   d. procedure used to dislodge airway obstruction

42. _____ supine   a. sitting up in bed

43. _____ Fowler's position   b. stomach lying

44. _____ foot drop   c. back lying

45. _____ prone   d. heel cord contracture

46. _____ void   a. shortening or tightening of muscle or tendon

47. _____ defecate   b. pass stool

48. _____ axillary   c. underarm

49. _____ cyanotic   d. bluish discoloration

50. _____ contracture   e. pass urine

Multiple choice (circle one correct answer)

51. An environment that is best for bacteria growth is one that is...

    a.   cool and dry
    b.   warm, moist and dark
    c.   brightly lit and hot
    d.   hot and dry

52. The average asymptomatic (no sign, no symptoms) period of time for HIV is...

    a.   3 months
    b.   2 years
    c.   10 years
    d.   6 months

53. Two blood borne pathogens are...

    a.   TB and HBV
    b.   HBV and UTI's
    c.   HBV and HIV
    d.   CPR and NPO

54. Oral care for the unconscious resident must be done...

    a.   Q 30 min.
    b.   BID
    c.   QID
    d.   Q 2 hours

55. Bath water temperature should not exceed...

    a.   120°
    b.   105°
    c.   96°
    d.   80°

56. When doing CPR, 30 compressions are followed by...

    a.   10 respirations
    b.   4 respirations
    c.   1 respiration
    d.   2 respirations

57. An environment that is helpful to the dementia resident is one that is...

    a.   loud, noisy and active
    b.   safe, quiet, gentle and reassuring
    c.   provides constant stimulation

58. An orange stick is used...

    a. to clean under the nails of the resident
    b. to use as a toothpick
    c. to use as a meat thermometer
    d. to help with positioning

59. When dressing a left hemiplegia resident in a sweater...

    a. put the left arm in the sleeve first
    b. put the right arm in the sleeve first
    c. it does not matter which arm you put in the sleeve first

60. Which type of resident is more likely to develop a decubitus ulcer?

    a. well nourished, ambulatory resident
    b. poorly nourished, paralyzed resident
    c. confused, ambulatory resident

61. What are signs of the first stage of a decubitus ulcer?

    a. open, draining wound
    b. pink, firm skin
    c. reddened area over a bony prominence

62. 8 oz. = _____ cc's

    a. 80 cc's
    b. 240 cc's
    c. 300 cc's
    d. 64 cc's

63. The urinary catheter bag should be placed...

    a. below level of bladder
    b. above level of bladder
    c. same level of bladder

64. 1000 cc = _____

    a. two quarts
    b. ¼ quart
    c. 1 quart

65. Low sodium diet means one that is low in...

    a. nutrients
    b. roughage
    c. pepper
    d. salt

66. Normal pulse rate is _____ per minute.

    a. 60-100
    b. 40-50
    c. 20-40
    d. 100-120

67. Peri care means cleaning the...

    a. feet
    b. ears
    c. face
    d. genital area

68. Proper body mechanics means that you should...

    a. twist your back when turning
    b. keep your back straight and bend at the knees
    c. bend at the waist

69. If the resident is paralyzed on their right side, which side should you place the chair that you will be transferring the resident to?

    a. left side
    b. right side
    c. it doesn't matter

Fill in the blanks with the correct answer.

List the grieving stages as described by Dr. Elizabeth Kubler-Ross.

70. _____

71. _____

72. _____

73. _____

74. _____

75. Elastic hose are prescribed by the physician to help prevent...

_____

76. Describe how you can warm a bottle of lotion before applying it to the resident.

_____

Name 3 bony prominences

77. _____

78. _____

79. _____

Explain what a progressive self feeding program is.

80. _____

List 2 symptoms of an impaction

81. _____

82. _____

The following questions pertain to CPR. Fill in the blanks.

83. Open the a _ _ _ _ _ by doing a head tilt, chin lift.

84. An unresponsive person doesn't move, makes no sound, and is not b _ _ _ _ _ _ _ _.

85. If the heart is not beating, there is no c _ _ _ _ _ _ _ _ _ _ _.

86. D _ _ _ _ _ _ _ _ _ _ _ _ _ _ means to deliver a shock to the heart by AED, to hopefully convert the heart to a normal rhythm.

List 2 possible causes of aggressive behavior by the resident.

87. _____

88. _____

Describe 2 observations about stool that should be reported to the charge nurse.

89. _____

90. _____

Describe 1 specific aging change associated with each of the following...

91. skin _____

92. digestive system _____

93. muscles _____

94. vision _____

95. cardiovascular _____

Describe two specific instances when gloves should be worn on the job.

96. _____

97. _____

Name three instances on the job when you must wash your hands.

98. _____

99. _____

100. _____

A

A.M. Care, 147
Abdominal trusts, 85, 86
Abduction, 238
Abraham Maslow, 21
Abuse, 12, 20, 33
Abusive behavior, 33
Acceptance, 258
Accident / incident report, 76
Accidents, 75
Acquired immunodeficiency syndrome, 133
Active range of motion, 238
Activities of daily living, 147
Adaptive self feeding devices, 190, 189
Adaptive/assistive devices, 233
Adduction, 238
Advanced directives, 258
Aggressive behavior, 24, 34, 251
Aging changes, 27
AIDS, 133, 135, 139
Airborne precautions, 124
Airway, 83
Airway obstruction, 85
Alarm cushion, 95
Alarms, 94
Alignment, 90
Alzheimer disease, 244, 247
Ambulation, 113, 218, 236
    ambulation equipment, 114
Amputation, 164, 272
Anger, 257
    anger-reducing tips, 34
Angina pectoris, 81
Antibodies, 134, 135
Anti-embolism stocking, 264
Aphasia, 43, 277
Apical pulse, 181
Appetite, 190
Applying lotion, 155, 165
Apraxia, 245
Asepsis, 127
    aseptic techniques, 120
Asphyxiation, 76
Aspiration, 157, 188, 190, 193
Assault, 13
Asymptomatic, 123
Atrophy, 232, 235, 237
Aural, 173
Axillary temperature, 176, 173

B

Back health, 101
Back injury, 100
Back rubs, 154, 259
Bacteria, 120, 121
Bacterial pneumonia, 274
Balance scale, 265
Bargaining, 258
Basic human needs, 21

Bathing, 148, 149
Battery, 13
Bed bolster, 95
Bedmaking, 225
Bedpan, 207, 206, 223
Bedside stand, 223
Behavioral disturbances, 244
Biohazardous waste, 125
Bladder, 205, 208
    bladder re-training program, 213
Bland diet, 188
Blindness, 272
Blocks to communication, 40
Blood borne pathogens, 118, 133, 142
Blood clot, 232, 264
Blood pressure, 178
Blood pressure cuff, 179
Body alignment, 110, 168
Body mechanics, 102
Bony prominences, 96, 151, 166
Bowel, 215
    bowel control training program, 218
    bowel elimination, 216
    bowel movement, 216, 218
Brachial, 181
    brachial artery, 180
Brain attack, 275
Breach of confidentiality, 140
Bronchitis, 273
Brushing teeth, 156
Burns, 76

C

Calibrated, 179
Call signal, 100, 222, 224, 259
Cane, 114
Carbohydrates, 186
Cardiac arrest, 81, 82
Cardiopulmonary resuscitation (CPR), 83
Carotid pulse, 80, 83, 181
Cast, 267
Catastrophic reactions, 245, 250
Catheter care, 209, 211
Center for Disease Control, 123, 140, 143
Centigrade, 173
Cerebrovascular accident (CVA), 275
Certified, 2
Charge nurse (RN), 234
Chemical restraints, 90, 91
Chest compressions, 83
Cheyne-stokes breathing, 259
Choices, 25, 252
Choking, 76, 85, 86
Cholesterol, 84
Chronic obstructive pulmonary disease (COPD), 273
Circulation, 111, 259
    circulatory system, 27
Cirrhosis of liver, 143
Clean, 128
Clean catch, 263

Foot care, 163
Foot drop, 94, 112, 235, 240
Footrests, 94, 108, 109, 112
Footwear, 113
Force fluids, 199
Fowler's position, 111, 259, 266, 271, 274
Fracture, 270
Fracture pans, 207
Friction, 167
Full fluids, 188

G

Gait belt, 75, 103, 104, 109, 113
Gangrene, 164
Gastrointestinal tract and digestion, 215
Gastrostomy tube, 194
Gatch handle, 222
Geri chair, 90
Glass non-mercury thermometer, 173
Gloves, 100, 122, 124, 125, 127
Good hygiene, 122
Good skin condition, 110
Gowns, 126, 127, 229
Graduate, 199
Grievances or disputes, 15
Grieving, 257
Grooming, 214
Gurney, 110

H

Half rails, 92
Hallucinations, 245, 249
Hand roll, 236, 240
Hand splint, 236
Handling linen, 229
Handwashing, 122, 127, 128
Hazards of immobility, 232
Health care acquired infections, 120
Health care team, 9
Hearing aids, 43
Heart attack, symptoms of, 82
Heart disease, 84
Heel cord contracture, 235
Heel/elbow protectors, 168
Height, 266
Helper T cells, 134, 135
Hemiplegia, 275, 276
Hepatitis A, 142
Hepatitis B, 123, 142
Hepatitis C, 143
Herniated disc, 101
Hierarchy of needs, 21
Hip flexion contractures, 235
Hip fracture, 74
   hip fracture surgery, 112
   hip pinning, 112

HIV, 123, 135
   HIV and drug use, 138
   HIV testing, 134
   HIV/AIDS, 133
   human immunodeficiency virus, 133
Housekeeping, 122
Hoyer lift, 102, 103, 104, 105, 265
Hyperalimentation or total parenteral nutrition, 194
Hypertension, 84, 178
Hypotension, 178

I

Ileostomy, 219
Illusions, 249
Immobility, 232
Immune system, 120, 133, 135
Immunity, 118
Immunizations, 122
Impaction, 216, 217, 232
Incontinence, 212
Indwelling (Foley) catheter, 209
Infectious agent, 122
Infectious materials, 128
Injury, 270
Insulin, 272
Insulin-dependent diabetes (type I), 272
Intake, 199
   intake and output, 199
Integumentary system, 30
Intermittent catheter, 210
Intravenous (I.V.) Feedings, 193
Invasion of privacy, 13
Ischemia, 166

J

Jobst stockings, 264

K

Kaposi's sarcoma, 141
Kidneys, 205,206

L

Labile moods, 277
Large intestine, 215
Laundry, 127
Left hemiplegia, 276
Legal considerations, 12
Legal ethical issues, 139
Lemon-glycerin swabs, 260
Licensed practical nurse (LPN), 8
Linen hampers, 127, 229
Linen handling guidelines, 127
Liver, 142

Answers to Quizzes, Homework, and Review

Chapter 1, pgs. 16-171.
1. a
2. c
3. c
4. a
5. true
6. true
7. false
8. false
9. true
10. Dispense medications, perform sterile technique procedure (see p. 7 for additional answers)
11. Physical therapist - works on strengthening muscles and helping resident regain mobility and ambulation
Occupational therapist - helps resident regain independence in ADL's (see pgs. 9 & 10 for additional answers)
12. Expose only the part of the body you are bathing, knock before entering room, maintain confidentiality of records and personal information (see pg. 14 for additional answers)
13. Check with your charge nurse

Chapter 2, pgs. 36-37
1. true
2. false
3. false
4. false
5. true
6. true
7. true
8. d
9. a
10. b
(For additional answers to questions #11 to #18 see pgs. 27-31)
11. Pumping efficiency of the heart decreases with decreased circulation to extremities
12. Decreased intestinal peristalsis
13. Decrease of muscle strength and agility
14. Lungs become more rigid and less flexible
15. Decreased bladder capacity and muscle tone
16. Decreased peripheral vision
17. Decreased hearing, especially of high-pitched sounds

18. More fragile skin
19. Encourage resident to be as mobile as possible, elevate their legs, keep their legs and feet warm, observe feet for possible complications such as sores that do not heal, avoid restrictive clothing
20. Possible death of spouse, possible increased isolation, increased health problems

Chapter 3, pgs. 52-53
1. a
2. b
3. c
4. c
5. d
6. Vision or hearing problems
7. Dementia
8. Fear
(see pg. 40 for additional answers to questions #6 to #8)
9. Skin tears
10. Rapid, labored breathing
11. Withdrawn behavior
12. Decreased appetite or inadequate fluid intake
(see pgs. 49-51 for additional answers to questions #9 to #12)
13. Resident complains of shortness of breath and a crushing discomfort in the chest, resident has fallen to the floor (there are other answers the instructor can discuss also)
14. Be patient and do not rush the resident , use gestures, pantomime, demonstrations and use of notepad and pencil. Use communication board and/or pictures. (see pgs. 43-44 for additional answers)
15. Speak clearly and concisely while facing the resident, communicate in an environment free of distractions, use non-verbal aids such as gestures, pantomime (see pg. 44 for additional answers)
16. false
17. true
18. false
19. false
20. false

Chapter 4, pgs. 71-72
1. Up as desired with bathroom privileges
2. Nothing by mouth after midnight until fasting blood sugar is done in the morning
3. 400 cubic centimeters by mouth, three times a day with meals
4. Up in wheelchair, assist with transfers as necessary
5. Take resident (patient) to physical therapy twice a day
6. Notify the nurse if the resident appears short of breath
7. Turn the resident every 2 hours with lotion rubs to the coccyx
8. Walk the resident with stand by assistance to the bathroom
9. Give good perineal care after incontinence
10. Range of motion to right upper extremity four times a day
11. Passive range of motion to left upper extremity twice a day
12. Obtain temperature, pulse and respiration and blood pressure and report to the charge nurse immediately
13. Encourage water intake to decrease chance of urinary tract infection
14. Check vital signs on resident immediately and every hour thereafter
15. Elevate head of bed on the resident with congestive heart failure
16. d
17. e
18. a
19. b
20. c
21. d
22. e
23. b
24. c
25. a

Chapter 5, pgs. 87-88
1. a
2. a
3. d
4. True
5. False
6. True
7. True
8. False

Answers to Quizzes, Homework, and Review

9. Spills on the floor, poor lighting, clutter (other examples on pg. 75)
10. Muscle weakness, paralysis, orthostatic hypotension.
11. Non-slippery shoes or slippers.
12. b
13. a
14. c
15. a
16. d
17. Pressure in chest, shortness of breath, pain that radiates to jaw, neck, shoulders, arms or back, nausea, (other symptoms listed on pg. 82).
18. To enable the breathing to be effective.
19. Inability to cough or speak, inability to breath.
20. Allow them to continue coughing until they are ok. Stand by to insure that it does not become a complete airway obstruction.

Chapter 6. pg. 98
1. a
2. a
3. c
4. d
5. Weaker muscles, increased agitation, increased pneumonia, cardiovascular stress (see pg. 91 for additional answers)
6. False
7. True
8. False
9. True
10. False

Chapter 7, pg. 115-116
1. False
2. False
3. False
4. False
5. True
6. False
7. False
8. True
9. Gait belt, Hoyer lift, slide boards, trapeze bars, draw sheets
10. Cervical - thoracic - lumbar
11. Disruption of the three natural curves which makes spine vulnerable to injury
12. Check environment for safety, evaluate your load, get close to your load, keep back straight, bend at the knees, ask

for help if necessary (see pgs. 102-103 for additional answers)
13. Obese residents, residents attached to tubes, residents with casts, residents who cannot bear weight on at least one good leg
14. any answer to question #13, if the resident has fallen to the floor, if you are unsure about your ability to transfer resident alone

Chapter 8, pgs. 130-131
1. True
2. True
3. True
4. False
5. False
6. True
7. False
8. False
9. False
10. True
11. Before and after resident contact, before putting on gloves and after removing gloves, after using bathroom (see pg. 128 for additional answers)
12. Handwashing, using gloves, using gowns and masks when necessary, sterilization and disinfection
13. c
14. b
15. b
16. d

Chapter 9, pgs. 144-145
1. False
2. True
3. True
4. True
5. False
6. True
7. True
8. True
9. Unprotected sex, sharing drug needles or syringes, engaging in high risk sexual behavior such as anal intercourse (see pg. 137 for additional answers)
10. Acquired immune deficiency syndrome
11. Human immunodeficiency virus
12. Kaposi's sarcoma
13. pneumocystis pneumonia
14. education, get tested, mutually monogamous sexual contact only with a person who

is not HIV positive (see pgs. 138-139 for additional answers)
15. Puncture wound with contaminated needle, blood splash to your mucous membranes
16. Fatigue, weight loss, nausea (see pg. 135 for additional answers)
17. Standard
18. isolation (see pg. 140 for additional answers)
19. Use standard precautions, practice "safer sex" techniques, get vaccinated

Chapter 10, pg. 170
1. False
2. False
3. True
4. False
5. False
6. True
7. True
8. True
9. True
10. True
11. c
12. Pressure, friction (see pg. 167 for additional answers)
13. Keep resident clean and dry, change resident's position at least every 2 hrs. (see pg. 168 for additional answers)

Chapter 11, pgs. 183-184
1. False
2. False
3. True
4. True
5. False
6. False
7. True
8. True
9. False
10. True
11. a
12. c
13. a
14. a
15. b
16. a
17. c
18. b

Chapter 12, pgs. 195-196
1. d
2. b
3. a
4. d
5. d
6. True

7. True
8. True
9. True
10. False
11. False
12. False
13. True
14. do not rush the resident at mealtime, position resident in an upright position during meal, resident to remain in upright position at least 20 minutes after eating (see pg. 193 for additional answers)
15. Plate with built up edges, rolling knife (see pg. 189 for other answers)
16. Quiet, calm, non-distracting environment. Give resident simple verbal cues to talk them through the feeding process.
17. Redness, swelling, bleeding, or complaints of pain

Chapter 13, pg. 203
1. False
2. True
3. True
4. True
5. False
6. True
7. 540 cc
8. 360 cc
9. 2 ml
10. Weakness, dry mucous membranes, confusion (see pg. 198 for additional answers)
11. Resident may have dysphagia, elderly people may lose their ability to feel thirst. Resident may not have ability to pour themselves fluids due to paralysis, weakness or confusion (see pg. 198 for additional answers)
12. b
13. c

Chapter 14, pgs. 219-220
1. False
2. True
3. True
4. True
5. False
6. True
7. False
8. True
9. False
10. False
11. b
12. c
13. d

14. a
15. e
16. a
17. d
18. b
19. c
20. b
21. Constipation means the resident can still pass stool although it is hard. Impaction means the resident cannot pass stool because it is so hard that it has created a blockage in the bowel

Chapter 15, pg. 230
1. True
2. False
3. True
4. True
5. True
6. False
7. False
8. True
9. False
10. d
11. b
12. c

Chapter 16, pgs. 241-242
1. b
2. b
3. a
4. ROM, use of hand roll, possibly a hand splint
5. ROM, use of foot rests to properly position the feet, use of foot board while in bed
6. Occupational therapist and nursing staff
7. Occupational therapist and nursing staff
8. Registered physical therapist, restorative therapy assistants and nursing staff
9. Built up spoon, plate guards, "sporks"
10. Velcro closures on clothing, a button hooker for a person who can only use one hand, long handled shoe horn
11. Paralyzed residents. Residents too weak to move on their own. Comatose or semi-comatose residents.
12. development of decubitus ulcer, muscle atrophy, pneumonia, osteoporosis (see pg. 232 for additional answers)
13. Encourage resident to move to their maximum ability and/or assist them to do so

14. Any redness, irritation or open area where the splint is applied

Page 254 Homework
1. A. It is important to recognize that he is upset and find out what is wrong. Once you know what is wrong you may be able to help.
2. C. It is important to recognize that the resident may be embarrassed about the incidence of incontinence. Attempt to work out a plan of toileting so this does not reoccur. Check with your charge nurse regarding a toileting plan.
3. There are numerous answers to this question. Some are: 1) Work with resident and her family on bringing objects and possessions which are meaningful to her to make her feel at home. Examples: photos, "favorite chair", afghan, personal items, etc. 2) escort resident to activity room, dining room, etc. and back to her room until she learns her way around. 3) Create a climate of acceptance and understanding. Allow resident to verbalize her feelings re. the recent losses in her life, i.e., husband, home, familiar surroundings.
4. Encourage resident to tell you about her career as a teacher and about her students. Redirect her to some meaningful activities she may enjoy. She may particularly like activities that involve children such as school groups that visit care centers, etc.
5. Bend down to resident's eye level and communicate with resident, even if you are not sure he can understand completely. Always tell him what you are going to do. Bring resident out of his room so he has a variety of environments during the day. Discuss with your charge nurse and activities director what may be appropriate activities for him. He may respond to music.

Chapter 17, pg. 255
1. True
2. False
3. False
4. True
5. True
6. True
7. True
8. False
9. False
10. True
11. b
12. e
13. d
14. d

Chapter 18, pg. 261
1. False
2. False
3. True
4. Do not resuscitate. A person does not wish to have CPR to resuscitate him/her.
5. Pre-written instructions on what life prolonging measures the resident may want.
6. to revive or bring back to life
7. after death care to the body
8. 1) Keep the resident clean and dry. 2) Maintain good position, which includes position change Q 2 hrs. 3) Respond quickly to resident's needs.

Chapter 19, pg. 268
1. False
2. True
3. False
4. False
5. True
6. a
7. b
8. d
9. 1) Report complaints of pain, tingling or numbness of limb in cast. 2) Report any wetness, odor or drainage from inside the cast 3) Check for signs of impaired circulation of the limb in the cast, such as fingertips or toes that are cool or cold to touch, bluish or purple and swollen
10. 1) Elevate head of the bed to Fowler's position. 2) Be supportive of resident since they may be anxious. Leave call light within reach of resident and check on her frequently.
3)Check for pressure on skin or discomfort possibly caused by nasal cannula.

Chapter 20, Pgs. 278-279
1. False
2. False
3. True
4. True
5. True
6. True
7. True
8. False
9. True
10. True
11. c
12. c
13. c
14. 1) Kidney disease 2)Amputations due to diabetic neuropathy 3) blindness due to retinopathy
15. 1) weakness or paralysis (right or left hemiplegia), assist resident as needed, encourage and assist efforts toward rehabilitation. 2) dysphagia, properly position resident at mealtimes and assist as needed. Be aware of dietary recommendations re. foods helpful for dysphagia.)3 aphasia, be patient and allow resident time to express self. Use gestures, pantomime, pictures, communication boards as necessary (see pgs. 277-278 for additional answers)

Review, pgs. 280-285
1. False
2. True
3. True
4. False
5. False
6. False
7. True
8. True
9. True
10. False
11. True
12. False
13. True
14. False
15. True
16. False
17. True
18. False
19. True
20. True
21. True
22. False
23. False
24. True
25. True
26. c
27. d
28. a
29. b
30. d
31. a
32. b
33. c
34. d
35. c
36. a
37. b
38. d
39. a
40. c
41. b
42. c
43. a
44. d
45. b
46. e
47. b
48. c
49. d
50. a
51. b
52. c
53. c
54. d
55. b
56. d
57. b
58. a
59. a
60. b
61. c
62. b
63. a
64. c
65. d
66. a
67. d
68. b
69. a
70. denial
71. anger
72. bargaining
73. depression
74. acceptance
75. edema
76. placing lotion bottle in basin of warm water or rub lotion in your hands to warm up
77. coccyx
78. hips
79. heels
80. supervised small group of residents who are gradually learning to feed themselves and are assisted as needed

81. absence of "normal" BM for several days
82. small, liquid smears of BM
83. airway
84. breathing
85. circulation
86. defibrillation
87. being fearful
88. loss of freedom of choice
89. black, tarry stool
90. hard stool
91. dry, fragile skin
92. decreased digestive enzymes
93. weaker muscles
94. impaired depth perception
95. takes longer for pulse to return to normal after period of stress
96. when potentially coming in contact with body fluids
97. when coming in contact with mucous membranes
98. between each resident
99. after removing gloves
100. after using bathroom